British Library Cataloguing in Publications Data

A catalogue record for this book is available from the British Library.

ISBN 978-0-9559361-3-5

Published by Assurance Publications Ltd,
The White House, Washington, NE37 1PG
United Kingdom

Tel: 07799653641

Email: info@assurancepublications.com
http://www.assurancepublications.com

Produced for Assurance Publications by Assurance Publishers
Cover Design and Content Design by
Kenteba Kreations
contact.kenteba@gmail.com

FOREWORD

It is with great honour that I write the foreword for this book "The Torch Bearer". I have known Dr. Elewechi Okike for over 30 years and what strikes me the most about her is the incredible journey of faith she has embarked on and her selfless life of serving others. Through the many trials and testings she has had to endure, she has stood on the infallible word of God, thereby remaining victorious in every way. There could not have been any more befitting title.

For many years she has inspired many, including myself with her exemplary life of pouring out to others. Her light has beamed even in the darkest hour.

There is nothing like a Kairos moment when Heaven intercepts Earth's agenda to cause a powerful encounter. Recognizing what I call a "God Moment", is when He is presenting an opportunity our way, and it is crucial to stepping into the next dimension of blessings that God has for us and His people.

The Torch Bearer is clearly a "God Moment". It was birthed out of a great and missed opportunity in the natural to be a Torch Bearer for the Olympics game. However through that experience, as disappointing as it may have seemed, a greater opportunity with a bigger impact was presented thereby seizing the moment.

Dr. Elewechi Okike has always lived a life by design; yes the life designed by God her Father. She strives to please the Father even in moments of uncertainty and uttermost difficulty. At a time of possible "lack of interest" in an event, it was all part of a grand design to bring about a greater and more dynamic glory for the Lord. As a Torch Bearer herself, her life's experiences are a culmination of encounters both bitter and sweet showing how a loving Father operates in our lives. "And we know that God causes everything to work together for the good of those who love God and are called according to his purpose for them" (Romans 8:28 NLT).

There is no question that this book:" The Torch Bearer" was ordained from the beginning. The God who is Alpha and Omega, the beginning and the end, worked the end of every experience shared in the book and retracted back to the beginning. This was so that Elewechi's testimony from series of journeys she has had to walk would become a light, touching and changing lives around the world. At the Olympics, a Torch Bearer at one point had been previously nominated and has gone through the process to eventually appear before the world bearing that Torch. There are specific paths they go through carrying that Torch and their goal is to successfully get to the appointed destination. Elewechi has met all of her life's challenges with such bravery, courage and faith. Just like the Olympics, she has been running the race and navigating the path that was set before her until she gets to her appointed destination. A Torch Bearer represents others from all walks of life. They are more or less an ambassador. She is indeed a Torch Bearer demonstrating the unwavering and unconditional love of God in the lives she touches. Through her publishing, charity work, career, devotionals, teachings and many other notable works she remains an ambassador of love, healing and recovery changing lives for the glory of God.

This book "The Torch Bearer" is a must read and could not have been written at a more significant season. It illuminates your mind and stirs you up to not only believe our Creator has a purpose but a destiny, a specific path for everyone small or great. As you take leaps of faith, He will enable you to do that which you cannot do on your own. The Torch Bearer provokes you to pay close attention to the moments of opportunity that are presented to you on a daily basis. With the leading of the Holy Spirit, He guides us into all truth.

God is looking for Torch Bearers who will say "Yes" I will go and be a light in dark places. God's light dissipates darkness and as demonstrated in the life of one Torch Bearer, you can make a difference. Out of the experiences you have been through, God begins to give you beauty for ashes, causing your testimonies to be a light of hope and encouragement to those you come in contact with. Would you be a Torch Bearer, willing to carry the flames of

His Love, hope and peace to your neighborhood, your community, your city, your state, country and ultimately the world?. The world needs more Torch Bearers who are willing to be lit and as you let His light shine through you, many will come to salvation, deliverance and restoration.

May you be blessed as your read this book and let the life changing experiences of this great vessel of God inspire you to become His "TORCH BEARER".

Dr. Chidi M. Kalu, Founder & President, Women of Distinction, Orlando Florida U.S.A.

PREFACE

**"We are called to bear His light
To a world where wrong seems right"**

(Steve Green – *People Need the Lord*)

We live in a world full of uncertainties, which can leave us with outcomes that can have life-changing consequences. Many of those who have read my book *The Greatest Debtor to His Love and a Trophy of His Grace,* no doubt arrived at the same conclusion as the BBC Tyne Reporter, Sarah Hathaway, who described my life as 'dramatic and eventful'. She made this remark after she had come to our home a second time, for a video interview with me. She confessed that she found some of my life's stories rather fascinating, and that if she had her way, she would come to our home again and again to do video interviews with me[1]. Indeed, the story of my life from my mother's womb has been quite dramatic. I count myself rather fortunate to still be alive in spite of some of the dramatic events in my life, many of which still make me shudder whenever I think of them. I recall a few people who when they were reading my book commented that the book had 'gripped' them. My neighbour said he felt like coming to knock on my door to ask what I had done to his wife; he could not get her attention anymore, as she was literally glued to my book. Of course, when the story of your life is so inspiring people want to read about it.

I hope that much more than *The Greatest Debtor,* readers of this new book, *The Torch Bearer* will find it even more inspiring. The title of the book itself tells the story. The idea for the book was conceived in 2012 following my nomination as one of the bearers

---

[1]See http://www.bbc.co.uk/tyne/content/articles/2007/09/28/tyne_abortion_video_feature.shtml, and http://www.bbc.co.uk/tyne/content/articles/2007/04/19/video_nation_escapefromslavery_video_feature.shtml .

of the Olympic Torch. When I started putting my thoughts together about the book, little did I know that another 'drama' was about to unfold in my life. The drama began when I woke up in the morning of Tuesday, October 9, 2012 and felt a lump on my right breast. Now that was real drama and I wish I could replay it again. As you read this book, you will discover a whole new world that has probably been alien to you. As more and more of this drama unfolded, I knew God allowed it for a purpose, and that He wanted me to write about my experience. Interestingly, most people really close to me confirmed what I had felt in my spirit. Many of them said to me 'don't worry; another book will come out of this experience'. I was now faced with the dilemma of what title I should give to my book. Should I write two separate books, one about the Olympic Torch and the other about life following a diagnosis of cancer? Not really! The Holy Spirit whispered to me that the story was one and the same. Whilst I was lamenting about missing a life time opportunity to be an Olympic Torch bearer, God was 'laughing' at me. It was as if He was saying to me 'daughter, you're missing the point here. I am not concerned about you not carrying the Olympic Torch, as important as you felt it was. It is about you being my Torch Bearer. I want you to show to the world how to shine my light in spite of the diagnosis of cancer. I want you to beam my light in a world where darkness seems to penetrate all strata of human existence'. Hence, the title of the book, *The Torch Bearer: Two Sides of the Story*.

I must say that it has been an emotional roller coaster putting down some of my experiences in this book. A few times I have found myself in tears all over again, as I have tried to recall some of my ordeal. My only consolation is that many who will read this book will find it to be truly inspirational, and appreciate what it is to be confronted with a diagnosis of a rare type of cancer, especially when it comes 'out of the blues'. More importantly, I pray that all who read this book will understand what it is to be a true *Torch Bearer*, whether in sickness or in health, one who would make an even greater impact in the lives of others than carrying the Olympic Flame would. Olympics do come and go, but the lives that we touch every day as we shine His light into the darkness in their lives will remain throughout eternity.

Elewechi Ngozi M. Okike

ABOUT THE BOOK ...

This is yet another spiritually inspired book by Dr Elewechi Ngozi Okike, about her experience of discerning the still small voice of our Sovereign Creator from the loud and sometimes noisy voices of the market place.

The Torch Bearer, is very well written, in the true African style of a story teller, which belies her African root and her in-depth knowledge of the word of God.

Dr Okike's research into the origin of the Olympic Games and the underlying spiritual implication, is yet, another challenge to Christians to heed the great Commission to: "Go ye into all the world and preach the gospel". We should proudly be the light of the world and go out in the market places of sports and our careers to proclaim to the world, how GREAT OUR GOD IS. It could also be through converting the Olympic sporting energy to Kingdom energy. The hymn writer wrote " SHINE JESUS SHINE.

Highly commendable work.

Sonny Iroche, CEO, Mutual Concepts Ltd, Lagos, Nigeria

This is a truly unique and moving book. It is one that takes the reader through a private and daunting journey which many make but almost always remains unspoken.

One enduring message which is summed up in this book, that even recent advances in medical science is not privy to, is the power of the human spirit; and how this relates to events of our life particularly in the outcome of difficult events.

Time and time again the writer stresses that she would not let her condition disrupt her life adversely or stop her life from normal activity. This is evidenced by her working right through the entire radiotherapy treatment and also having minimal reaction from the therapy. A general observation I made for quite some time now as someone who sees hundreds annually is that often you can tell those who will do well by their courage and fearless spirit. As a result, this book has ministered to me personally and also I am certain there is something unique there for all who read it.

Mr Obi Iwuchukwu, FRCS, FRCS(Gen), MD
Consultant Breast & Oncoplastic Surgeon, Sunderland Royal Hospital, UK

This is indeed a fascinating read; really arresting and life inspiring.

Dr Goke Aiyegbayo, MD Rickleton Medical Centre, Washington, UK

DEDICATION

To the glory of God this book is dedicated to all those men and women (doctors, nurses, family and friends) that God used to minister to me in one way or the other during the 'season' in my life discussed in this book. It is also dedicated to all those men and women whose lives will be touched and transformed through reading this book.

ACKNOWLEDGEMENTS

I would like to thank all those who have made it possible for me to write this book, especially my brother, Sonny, who nominated me to be one of the carriers of the Olympic Flame. If he had not done so, I would probably not have had the inspiration to write a book with such a title.

I also want to use this opportunity to express my gratitude to all those who stood by me and supported me and my family in so many ways, either through visits, phone calls, the provision of food and much more with their prayers, during what has been one of the most difficult and challenging periods in my life. Drs Onyebuchi and Pat Eseonu, Dr Myra Herbert, Dr John and Mrs Margaret Ameobi, Drs James and Betty Nwabineli, Dr Olamide Olukoga, Mr and Mrs Mode, Mr and Mrs Abladey, Margaret John, Mr Charles Uwakaneme, Dr Nsidinanya Okike, Mr Ogbonnaya and Rosemary Okike, Mr Steve and Mrs Vera Ailemen, Ms Temitope Fodunrin, Pastor and Mrs Bolaji Ismail, Mr Jonas and Mrs Comfort Abladey, Dr Francis and Mrs Amaka Ndaji, Chidi Kalu, Kalu Omokwe, Mr Sonny and Mrs Suzanne Iroche, Mr Cyril Asuquo, Mrs Christy Omoruan and many more too numerous to mention. Drs Onyebuchi and Pat Eseonu deserve special mention for the role they played in my life, and the support they gave to me and my family, and the sacrifice they made, financial and otherwise. May the Lord you have all honoured in the sacrifices that you made and the love that you showed, reward you mightily.

Special thanks also go to my GP, Dr Goke Aiyegbayo, the Consultant Surgeon, Mr Obi Iwuchukwu, the Macmillan nurse, Michelle Derbyshire and all the other doctors, nurses and radiographers that God used to take care of me. It is because of the role they played that I have a story to tell. They ensured that I received the best possible treatment, care and attention. I am indeed grateful for all their love, care and support.

Finally, I want to thank my immediate family for the role they have played in my life and for all the love, understanding and support they gave to me during this difficult time. My husband and children rose to the challenge, and were there for me any time.

God, my Father, deserves special thanks too, for leading me thus far in my walk with Him, teaching me to know how to turn the trials, challenges and obstacles that I face in my life into stepping stones that bring glory and honour to His name. He has taught me that carrying a physical torch is not as important as being His true Torch Bearer, in sickness and in health.

Special thanks to Joojo Kyei for the lovely design of the book cover and most of the art work. Thanks also to Uche Okike for the lovely photo (HUG in a Bag) used in the book.

I would also like to express my appreciation to all who took time to read the first draft of the book and provided me with valuable comments, suggestions and feedback, which have helped in refining the contents of the book – Mr Kalu Omokwe, Dr Chidi Kalu, Chief Sonny Iroche, Dr Goke Aiyegbayo, Mr Obi Iwuchukwu, and last, but not the least, my husband, Dr Chikezie Okike, and my daughter, sister and friend, Miss Adaeze Okike. The responsibility for the contents of the book remains mine.

CONTENTS

PART ONE
One side of the Story

PART TWO   -

The Other side of the Story

LIST OF ABBREVIATIONS

NKJV – New King James Version of the Bible
NIV – New International Version of the Bible
SRH – Sunderland Royal Hospital
MDT – Multi-disciplinary Team

(Note: All translations are from the NKJV of the Bible, unless otherwise specified.

PART ONE

ONE SIDE OF THE STORY

INTRODUCTION

The Olympics is the premier sporting event in the world of sports. Every true athlete has an ambition of winning a medal at an Olympic Game. As a matter of fact, winning a gold medal is often seen as 'the pinnacle' of the career of most athletes. It is an event which may take place at one's doorstep (home country) once in a life time. Many countries aspire to host the Games for a number of reasons, including the economic benefits of hosting the events.

On a personal level, I am not a sports enthusiast although I enjoy watching them on TV occasionally and that is as far as it would go. Being a wife and mother of three sons and one daughter, I live in a male-dominated home and so have found myself watching football on TV when it comes on. Moreover, our youngest son got very close to being a professional footballer, but it was not meant to be. However, as far as I was concerned, whether the Olympic Games were taking place in England or not, I was not really bothered. Visiting London outside of the Olympics was bad enough, much more doing so during the period of the Games. I told myself that nothing would take me to London during that period, even if I was offered free tickets to go and watch the Games. Given my perception about the event, it did not come as a surprise that when I was nominated as one of those to carry the Olympic Torch, a key symbol of the Games, I did not accept the nomination, even when a reminder was sent to me two months later. I did not even read the emails to find out more about what it entailed much less following up with an enquiry. The truth of the matter was that I was not interested.

On the 7th of November 2011, I was watching the news on the television in my kitchen whilst I was having my breakfast, and it was mentioned that the names of those who would be carrying the Olympic Flame across the country had been published. All of a sudden it dawned on me that I had missed an opportunity of a life-time. The Olympics do not come to your doorstep every day. I felt my whole body tremble. I was in shock. What have I done to myself? I was overcome by inexplicable grief.

There were three possibilities open to me when I was nominated: one was to accept the nomination and then not be picked in the final selection process. That being the case, the matter would have ended there and I would have consoled myself with the thought that at least I did make an effort. The second option was to accept the nomination, be successful in the selection process and then have the opportunity to carry the Olympic Flame. The third option, which I chose, was not to accept the nomination at all, but which opened my eyes and broadened my perspective on the whole symbolism of what it is to be a TORCH BEARER, which is what has inspired me to write this book. Out of what appeared to be a missed opportunity, something much more edifying has been birthed. Interestingly, none of the first two options would have inspired me to write this book. Even if following my nomination, I was selected to carry the Flame and chose to write a book about the experience, it would probably have a different slant to it.

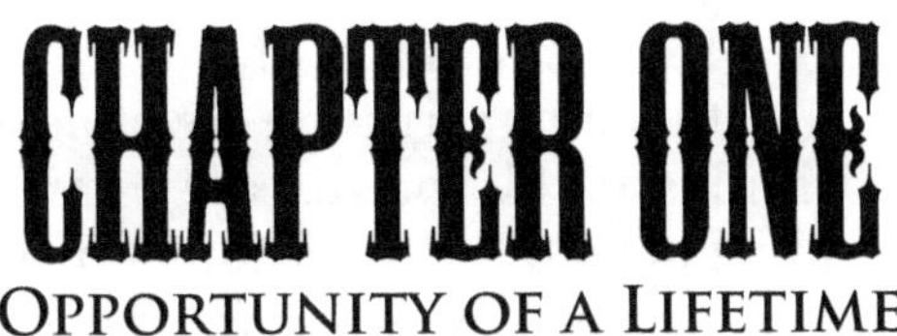

CHAPTER ONE
OPPORTUNITY OF A LIFETIME

Once in a while, life presents us with opportunities, but through ignorance and, or carelessness, we can allow such opportunities to pass us by. This was what happened to me during the London 2012 Olympic Games.

I had been nominated in July by my brother, Sonny, a good customer of Lloyds TSB, one of the companies at the forefront of promoting the Games. I did not bother to read the email to find out what was required to be an Olympic Torch bearer. In my ignorance, I had assumed that one would need to be fit and strong and have to travel to London to carry the torch. Both assumptions were wrong and unfounded. Although in my correspondence with my brother, I had indicated that I would make further enquiries about it, I never did. I simply forgot to do so. I think I got too busy with other things that I felt were more important to me.

In September 2011, I received another reminder email from my brother, being one he had received from his bank saying that his nominee was yet to accept his nomination. As a matter of fact, I was taken aback when I received this reminder email. It was as if fate was knocking on my door, and trying to give me another opportunity of a life-time – to carry the Olympic Flame. Would there ever be another Olympics in England in my lifetime? In my busy schedule, I had completely forgotten about this nomination, and it was good to discover that the opportunity was still there for me to make some effort to find out more about what carrying the Torch would entail. Still, I did nothing about it. Then when I heard the news on television that the names of those that would carry the Olympic Flame had been released, it dawned on me that I had missed an opportunity of a life-time - to carry the Torch, which for me would have been a symbol of carrying the LIGHT OF THE GOSPEL, across this nation. It was the spiritual symbolism or significance that hit me the most. My whole body trembled.

I remember telling what I had heard in the news. He said "you don't have to be an athlete to carry the Olympic Torch. After all, Mohammed Ali with his Parkinson disease carried it". It dawned on me again that I had missed the opportunity of a life-time. In my ignorance I thought such an activity was reserved for athletes, who were physically fit, and able to run with the torch. I do not have such stamina, I thought. He said I should not flog myself, but let it go. "It has happened and there's nothing you can do about it", he said.

I fell on my knees and cried out to God, to forgive me for not even praying about it, when I received the emails. I did not bother to read about it, to find out more, which was very unlike me. I felt totally helpless and needed someone to pray with me. My husband had already gone out, so I went into our son's room to see if he was there. He was trying to get out of his bed, and noticing how distressed I was, he asked what was wrong. This made him jump out of bed immediately. Thank God he's a young man whose heart is seriously after God, and so he could understand when I tried to tell him what had happened and how I was feeling. We started praying, and I could not stop crying. I was heart-wrenched! I felt I had let God and my family down. How could I have missed such an opportunity?

We talked about a lot of things happening with us individually and collectively, and the fight against destiny killers. We spent some time praying together. There was a word my son used when he was praying that hit me. He prayed that God would <u>MAGNIFY</u> His voice above all other voices that we hear, so that we would always be sure to be in the centre of His will. I thought that was profound. If I did not have appointments at work that day, I would have worked from home, because my head ached badly, from all the crying, and the fact that I had worked late into the night.

I managed to get to work, though my head pounded very badly. Strangely, I did not get out of work till about 8.45pm, even though my last appointment for the day was at 6.30pm. When our daughter rang me that evening on her way from work, holding my head with one hand, I told her about my ordeal. She also tried to console me, saying 'don't worry, mum, these things happen'. I took some pain killers and Camomile tea and went to bed earlier than normal, at 11.30pm.

As I lay in bed in the early hours of the next day, I could not help thinking about this Olympic Torch matter. I rolled out of bed to pick up my Laptop to look through the emails I had received from my brother to refresh my memory on our correspondence on this issue. I could not believe that the nomination was as far back as July. The first email was dated 28th July 2011. I recall that after I received this email informing me about the nomination, my reply was "My brother, thanks for the nomination. I don't think I'm in the position to carry the Olympic Torch as I don't live in London and have no plans to attend any of the events. I'll pass on this one". His reply was "Ok, I thought the torch carrying would be in your locality. I understand if you turn it down. But it's a positive thing if it's in your neighbourhood". I then replied "I'm not so sure if there'll be torch carrying in our area. I thought it was restricted to London. If there is, of course, it'll be good publicity, and I wouldn't mind giving it a try. I'll make enquiries and see how it goes". I was actually on my way to the post office to post my brother's letters to him in London. After I got back, I never followed up on our discussion. I forgot about it again.

I travelled to South Africa and Ghana (that is a testimony of its own!) between 30th August and 11th September. One of the emails that I received on my return was one sent on the 9th of September, from my brother. He had received it from his bank and forwarded it to me. The subject was "Your nominee still needs to accept their Torchbearer nomination", and it read

"Hi Sonny,

You nominated Elewechi Okike to be a Torchbearer in the London 2012 Olympic Torch Relay with Lloyds TSB. The **deadline is fast approaching** and Elewechi has not yet accepted the nomination.

Now would be a great time to encourage Elewechi to accept and complete the process.

Due to high demand in the last days of the campaign we've extended the deadline for nominees to accept their nomination, but it must close at **11.59pm on Monday 26 September.**

Don't forget, if you're a Lloyds TSB Customer, once your nominee has accepted the nomination we'll enter you into a prize draw, giving you a chance to win a pair of tickets to London 2012 – another great reason to make sure your nominee accepts!

Good luck!
The Lloyds TSB Olympic Torch Relay Team"

When I read the email, I was quite surprised, and exclaimed "what! this thing is still there?" It appeared to me that the Relay Team was more desperate than I was. And come to think of it; the deadline for accepting nominations was extended, yet I never bulged. What a pity!

I had forgotten what I had written in my earlier correspondence with my brother, that I would be making enquiries about it. So, as the reality of it all hit me as I lay on my bed, I went back to look at all the emails. In fact, when I realised that if I accepted his nomination, my brother would have had the opportunity to be entered into a prize draw to win a pair of tickets for the London 2012 Games that even broke me the more.

Although I was nominated to carry the Olympic Flame, it did not necessarily imply that I would have been selected. Nevertheless, at least I would have given myself the opportunity to be picked, and my conscience would have been clear.

I suppose the reality of it all was hitting me so hard, that I eventually decided to go into 'Google' to find out more about the Olympic Torchbearer, and saw a section headed "Olympic Flame's 8,000-Mile route Revealed". It said the torch will be taken within an hour's journey of 95 percent of the population as it passes through 1,018 villages, towns and cities". It also read 'on parts of the journey, torchbearers will carry the flame on horseback, by bicycle, tram and steam train ... the 70 day relay will start at Land's end in Cornwall on the morning of May 19. It then travels an estimated 8,000 miles around the UK carried by 8,000 torchbearers, each picked because of a 'PERSONAL ACHIEVEMENT or CONTRIBUTION TO THE LOCAL COMMUNITY'. Now, that hit me really hard, as I realised why my brother had nominated me. To make matters worse, I read further to find out which areas will be covered and it included Newcastle, Lowfell, Gateshead, Sunderland, etc. Again, it dawned on me that I had missed an opportunity to carry the Torch, which for me would have symbolized carrying the flame of God's love around my community and shining for Jesus.

Incidences like this do not just happen. It was very unlike me not to have opened my brother's email to read the details, and to follow up the enquiries as I had mentioned, knowing that it would have provided me with the opportunity to talk about the work that I am doing with Book Aid for Africa (BAFA)(www.bookaidforafrica.com), and perhaps to also share my faith. I suppose I shunned it all because I was only thinking about me, and not wanting to draw attention to myself, which of course is what Matthew 6: 1-4, says – *"Be careful not to perform your good works publicly to be noticed by people; else you forfeit reward from your Father who is in heaven. Thus, when you give charity, do not blow a trumpet ahead of you as the hypocrites do in the synagogues and in the streets to gain glory from men. I assure you, they have reward. But when you practice charity, your left hand must not know what your right is doing, so that your charity will be in secret. And your Father who sees in secret will reward you"* (Modern Language version).

However, beyond that, God used the incident to speak to me very strongly, as I spent time in prayer trying to unravel this mystery. Here are some of the things the Holy Spirit spoke to me:

1. I must always see God's perspectives in everything. It is never about me, but about Him!

2. I must PRAY and ask God about everything I want to embark on, including things that I do not understand until He gives clarity.

3. The sin of 'omission' is as bad as the sin of 'commission'. When we neglect to do what God asks us to do, or disobey Him in fully carrying out His instructions, we are equally guilty.

4. He has allowed this for a purpose to teach me some important lessons about "recognising the day of God's visitation". Olympics do not come everyday!

5. He has removed the veil over my eyes. Although, I hear from

Him in my daily walk with Him, I will hear Him much more.

6. I will learn to trust Him more, and take GIANT STEPS OF FAITH, and know that 'with Him, all things are possible".

7. It is not always good to shy away from recognition. I have done it before, and it cost me dearly (but God still turned it around for good). It is God that honours, and not man.

In the chapters that follow, I expand on some of these truths.

I prayed and asked God to forgive me if in any way, I missed walking through a door which He Himself opened for me. He is rich in mercy and compassion. I know He forgave me, even though at the time it was very hard for me to forgive myself. Knowing that "all things work together for the good of those who love God", I got really excited about the good thing that would come out of what appeared to me at the time to be a missed opportunity.

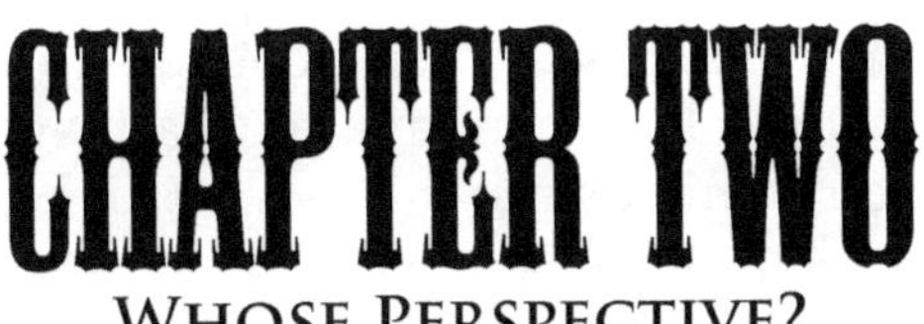

CHAPTER TWO
WHOSE PERSPECTIVE?

Quite often, when we look at things from our own perspective, we can make the wrong decisions or arrive at wrong conclusions. It is sometimes necessary to step back and to see the bigger picture. Most importantly, we need to ask ourselves, what does God think about this? Or who would benefit, or be disadvantaged, from this action that I am about to take?

One of the reasons why I was reluctant to accept my nomination as an Olympic Torch Bearer was because I was only looking at it from my own perspective. I did not want any unnecessary publicity for myself. The media reported that "8,000 inspirational people from around the UK will carry the Olympic Flame as it journeys across the UK. Nominated by someone they know, it will be their moment to shine, inspiring millions of people watching in their community, in the UK and worldwide". Did I really want to shine that way? I was only thinking about ME, and no other person. Perhaps if I had taken time to reflect on how my participation would have benefitted others, the outcome would have been different.

Firstly, carrying the Olympic Torch would have had a spiritual significance for me, as a Christian. In Matthew 5: 14, the Bible declares *"You are the light of the world. A city built on a hill cannot be hidden"* (Modern Language version). Running 300 metres with that Flame would have reminded me of that injunction in Matthew 5: 16 *"Don't hide your light! Let it shine for all; let your good deeds glow for all to see, so that they will praise your heavenly Father"* (Living Bible).

Secondly, as we all watched the events and activities planned before, during and after the Torch Relay in different parts of the country, it was obvious that it was more than just carrying the Flame. The Olympic Flame lit up whole communities figuratively speaking. Friends and families came out to cheer their heroes and it was a proud moment for all who were connected with the Torch

Bearers. I was particularly sad when I noticed from the route map for the Flame that my local community, Washington, was not on the list. I reasoned within myself that perhaps if I had accepted my nomination, I would have helped to put my local community on the map. This made me feel like I had let my whole community down, not just my family and friends. They would all have been so proud of me.

Thirdly, I did not give due consideration to the reason why I was nominated in the first place, to be a Torch Bearer. My brother who nominated me was aware, and truly proud, of the work I was involved in, Book Aid for Africa (BAFA)[2], a Charity that I established in 2007, that is making a difference in the educational landscape in different parts of Africa. Besides, it is helping to provide work placement opportunities for locals in the community. Being nominated and selected to carry the Flame would have provided a unique opportunity to promote the work of the Charity, more so, as we are in dire need of funds to ship books to Africa.

Indeed, looking at my nomination as an Olympic Torch Bearer from my perspective only, had outcomes that in retrospect, I would not have chosen. I missed the opportunity to be God's ambassador, carrying the flame of His love across my community and promoting a good cause that is making a difference in the lives of others.

I must always see God's perspectives in everything. It is never about me, but about Him! Perhaps if I thought more about the spiritual symbolism or significance of carrying the Torch as an ambassador for God's kingdom, I would have taken the necessary steps to do what I needed to do.

---

[2]See www.bookaidforafrica.com

CHAPTER THREE
DON'T BE PRESUMPTUOUS

I cannot recount how often I have suffered loss, heartache and pain as a result of presumptuousness. When one is presumptuous, one takes so much for granted. Some ideas may be good, but are they God's ideas? This is why we must always step back and pray before we embark on any course or action.

Prayer is our link to God. It helps us to find out what we should or should not do, especially when we are confronted with destiny shaping decisions. We must PRAY and ask God about everything we want to embark on, including things that we do not understand until He gives us the go ahead. In my case, if I had prayed and asked God whether or not I should accept my nomination, I probably would not have felt so bad. I think my not praying about it made me feel even worse.

The Bible presents us with many examples of people who prayed until they received clear guidance and direction from God. One of such people was King David. In 1Samuel 23: 2, we read *'Then they told David, saying, Behold, the Philistines fight against Keilah, and they rob the threshing floors. David ASKED THE LORD, "shall I go and attack them?" "Yes, go and save Keilah," THE LORD TOLD HIM'*. When his men were afraid to go and fight the Philistines, we are told (verse 4) that *'David ASKED THE LORD AGAIN, and the Lord again replied, "Go down to Keilah, for I will help you conquer the Philistines"*. With this assurance, David went ahead and did conquer the Philistines.

We can always be assured of a positive outcome, when we follow God's leading and guidance. On this occasion we find that David even asked the Lord TWICE, to make assurance doubly sure. Also in 1Samuel 30 we find that when David and his men returned from battle and arrived at Ziklag, the Amalekites had destroyed the city with fire and taken away all the women and children, including David's two wives, Ahinoam and Abigail. David and the people who were with him were so distraught that they cried out to God until they had no more strength left in them. The people even wanted to kill David because of all that had happened to them. Instead of taking the law into his own hands and running after the Amalekites, we are told that '*David ASKED THE LORD, "Shall I chase them? Will I catch them?" And the Lord TOLD HIM, "Yes, go after them; you will recover everything that was taken from you!"* (Living Bible verse 8). And it was so; David went after them and recovered everything, including the women and children who had been taken captive.

When we presumptuously take steps outside of God's direction, the consequences can be quite devastating, as it was for me. David also discovered this truth. In 2Samuel 24 we read about how David presumptuously went ahead and numbered the children of Israel and Judah, without him asking, or seeking clearance from God. And after he did it, his heart condemned him (verse 10), and he cried out to God. This action of David brought about disastrous consequences for the children of Israel and Judah. God sent a great plague amongst them such that seventy thousand people died in one day. Is it not amazing to find that a man like David who understood the secret of always asking God before taking action could go ahead and number the people when God did not tell him to do so. Perhaps this is why he prayed in Psalm 19: 12-13 "*Who can understand his errors? Cleanse me from secret faults. Keep back your servant from presumptuous sins; let them not have dominion over me. Then I shall be blameless, and I shall be innocent of great transgression*" (NKJV).

CHAPTER FOUR
OMISSION OR COMMISSION

The sin of 'omission' is equally as bad as the sin of 'commission'. When we neglect to do what God asks us to do, or disobey Him in fully carrying out His instructions, we are equally guilty.

When we commit the sin of omission, we fail to do what is expected of us. How many times do we receive emails and, or text messages which we fail to reply? Sometimes, a short and simple reply is all that might be required to ward off a misunderstanding. Many of us expect to receive a reply when we send an email or text message. But sometimes, we do to others what we would not like others to do to us – ignore their emails or text messages. This is not suggesting that every email or text message requires a response. As a matter of fact, there are some of them that you are better off not replying to, and I have personally received a few of those. However, this was definitely not the case in relation to my nomination to carry the Olympic Flame.

After our initial exchange of correspondences, I did indicate to my brother, that I would give the nomination a try, especially after I had received the reminder in September 2011. The email did require a response; accept or decline (after praying about it, of course); yet I could not get myself to simply click on the reply button to accept or decline my nomination. Instead, I did nothing; but simply got too busy, or remained indifferent about it.

Whereas with the sin of omission, we know what we should do, but we fail to do it; with the sin of commission, we actually know the right thing to do but choose to do otherwise. The right thing I should have done when I received the reminder email in September was to accept or decline my nomination. Instead I did the wrong thing, which was not to reply, or to ignore the emails. I am not exactly sure that I deliberately chose not to reply. I think I simply got carried away with doing other things that I did not make a note of the closing date for accepting nominations. On the other hand, if it was important to me, I would probably not have delayed replying. Some other person would have been very excited about the nomination that they would not think twice about it, but would simply reply. We are talking about the Olympics here, and an opportunity to be on the world stage, and listed amongst those who carried the Olympic Flame in the history books. How could anyone be indifferent about such an opportunity?

I felt really bad to have let my brother down; and not only himself, but my family and friends. Sometimes I would close my eyes and imagine the excitement of family and friends, especially my grand-children, to see their nana running with the Olympic Flame. I am pretty sure I would have taken a few shots with them, and it would probably have been the proudest moment of their lives. However, these were simply illusions. I did not give myself the opportunity for that to happen because through my carelessness I did not see the historic significance of carrying the Flame. It was not only a sin of omission on my part, but one of commission as well.

Most often, the sin of commission carries with it destiny shaping consequences. All through the Bible, from Genesis to Revelation, we read about how God dealt with people who disobeyed Him by choosing to do the wrong thing, when they knew the right thing to do. Today, the world is paying a very costly price for the disobedience of Adam and Eve in the Garden of Eden. They knew the right thing, which was not to eat the fruit in the midst of the Garden as they were instructed (Genesis 2: 16-17), yet they listened to the voice of the serpent, who deceived them, and in disobedience, ate the fruit (Genesis 3: 4-6). As a result, their relationship with God was severed. Thus through this simple act of disobedience, man has had a broken relationship with God. This relationship has thankfully been restored through the death and resurrection of Jesus Christ.

The simple definition of sin according to James 4: 17 is *"knowing what is right to do and then not doing it"* (Living Bible). Today, the sin of commission is having devastating consequences in the lives of men and women all over the world.

CHAPTER FIVE
Seize the Moment

One of the reasons why I think God allowed me to experience the devastation I felt when I failed to accept my nomination was to teach me some important lessons about knowing how to seize the moment, when opportunities present themselves. Christians would explain it as "recognising the day of God's visitation". The Olympics do not come every day! In fact, when they do, they are not always at your doorstep. Many people who knew this made the most of the opportunity. A lot of businesses flourished, and many became very rich as a result of the Olympics being held in England. As a matter of fact, those towns and cities that were on the routes for the Torch Relay were completely transformed. Lots of activities and events were held just to commemorate the arrival of the Olympic Flame.

Many people do miss their blessings in life by failing to seize the moment; to recognise God-given opportunities and to make the most of them. I think that was what happened to me. I was so completely ignorant and perhaps indifferent about the whole Olympics that I failed to see it as an opportunity not just to be part of history, but much more, to promote the Charity, for which I was nominated in the first place. I did not seize the moment.

All through the Bible we read about people who knew how to seize the moment when the opportunity presented itself. One of such people was Blind Bartimeus, the son of Timaeus, who sat by the roadside begging (Mark 10: 46-52). He heard that Jesus of Nazareth was passing by with His disciples and a great multitude following Him. It was an opportunity that Blind Bartimeus would not miss, even if he had to scream at the top of his voice. Nothing was going to stop him; though the people tried to shut him up. That action made him shout so much more. And guess what? Jesus of Nazareth, heard him, and stopped. Can you imagine the scenario? This man got Jesus' attention because he was prepared to seize the moment. Jesus asked him what he wanted, and his answer was (Mark 10: 51), *"Master, let me receive my sight"* (Revised Standard Version). Did he receive what he asked for? Of course he did. If that blind man did not seize that moment that presented itself, he would probably have remained blind for the rest of his life.

The other fascinating story in the bible about people who knew how to seize the moment, is that of the woman with the issue of blood (Mark 5: 25-34). This woman had suffered hemorrhages for 12 years and had spent all her money paying doctors to cure her of her ailment, but rather than getting better, her condition grew worse. Jesus was on his way to the house of Jairus, whose daughter was at the point of death. A large crowd was following Jesus, but there was someone who had made up her mind that she was not just going to be part of a crowd. Here was an opportunity too good to miss. She had her strategy well mapped out – just to touch "*the hem of His garment*", even if it meant squeezing herself through the crowd. As she did that, her hemorrhage ceased, and Jesus knew that someone had made a demand on His power; someone had touched Him in a way that was significant. Jesus sought to identify the person and the woman presented herself, and told Jesus her story. Jesus admired her courage and fortitude. The woman received her healing. If she had allowed the size of the crowd to put her off, or what people would think of her, she would probably have remained with her hemorrhage for the rest of her life, which could have led to her death.

I am not usually a TV enthusiast; however, my favourite TV shows are the talent shows. And one of the reasons why I like them is because of the opportunity they give to ordinary people, who are willing to seize the moment. Today many celebrities have emerged from 'Britain's Got Talent', X-Factor, 'Voice UK', etc. These are people who were willing to seize the moment when the opportunities presented themselves. If they just stayed home to watch others on the TV, they would not be enjoying all the fame and recognition, and of course the money that goes with it, too.

Besides celebrities, many successful people in the world today are in that position because they were able to recognise, and to cease the moment, when opportunities presented themselves. It is possible for two friends to go on holiday to China or India, or to some other country. One of them might see the trip as just another holiday, whilst the other who understands what it is to seize the moment, might see business opportunities, in addition to the holiday. A lot of this has to do with our mindset. If our way of thinking is geared towards a particular ideology or way of life, we might miss divine moments and fail to walk through doors which God might be opening up for us. My experience of not accepting my nomination as a Torch Bearer, and failing to seize the moment was a bitter pill to swallow.

There are many things that can stop one from 'seizing the moment' when opportunities present themselves. These include: procrastination; that is, putting off what should be done immediately, until later. In most cases, the things never get done. Another factor is the fear of what others might think. People who received their miracles like Blind Bartimeus and the woman with the issue of blood did not care about what anyone would have thought. They needed their breakthrough and that was all that mattered. Complacency and apathy are also factors that can stop people from taking action or seizing the moment when they should.

This notwithstanding, as Christians we must differentiate between seizing the moment and being opportunistic, or taking undue advantage of others, or of a situation. With the help of the Holy Spirit, we can always discern when God expects us to take action that would bless others.

CHAPTER SIX
MAGNIFY YOUR VOICE

In the 21ˢᵗ Century in which we live, there would appear to be many demands on our time, and we have all become extremely busy. Such busyness can make our lives so crowded with activities, that if we do not have good time management skills, we may not get our priorities right. We can even miss important deadlines, fail to take advantage of opportunities, or fail to reach specific goals and targets. I am not exactly sure whether that was the reason why I did not reply to the emails requesting me to accept my Torch Bearer nomination, or whether it was more to do with a lack of interest. However, I know that the reality of missing such an opportunity to be one of the Torch Bearers hit me very badly. I recall that in my deflated state, our youngest son prayed with me, and used an expression that drove an important message home. He prayed that in the midst of all the clutter and clatter in our lives, God would <u>MAGNIFY</u> His voice above all other voices that we hear, so that we would always be sure to be in the centre of His will. How so true!

Oftentimes when we are faced with important decisions, we find ourselves struggling within, and it would appear that we are hearing many voices at the same time trying to tell us which is the option we should choose. A sensible Christian would know that at such times it is best to do nothing, but to pray until God gives clear guidance. Someone would ask 'but how do I know it is God speaking to me?' Well, the answer is simple, God speaks to us in a 'still small voice', and usually, you will feel a sense of peace within. The inner struggles would cease. In Proverbs 20: 27, the Bible says *"the spirit of man is the candle of the Lord"*. Indeed, Jesus said in John 10: 27 *"My sheep recognize my voice, and I know them, and they follow me"*.

God also speaks to us through His word, as the Psalmist rightly declared (Psalm 119: 105): *"your word is a lamp unto my feet, and a light to lighten my path"*.

Some people feel comfortable asking friends and family for advice when they are confused and do not know which way to turn. There is nothing wrong with that. But the point is that we are all different, and what might seem to be the right course of action for one person, might not necessarily be the same for another person. It is sometimes even safer to make a decision first, and then have it validated by others. This does not mean we must change our minds if others do not agree with our decision. However, the bible says in 2Corinthians 13: 1 that *"in the mouth of two or three witnesses, every statement will be confirmed"* (Living Bible).

Perhaps following the example of Jesus is one way of dealing with the clutter in our lives. Many times we read that He always made out time to pray. After spending so much time with the multitudes that thronged Him daily, He would withdraw into a quiet place to 'recharge His batteries', so to speak. There is nothing as disastrous as trying to make a life-changing decision without taking sufficient time to reflect on the different options and outcomes. Many of us will recall times in our lives when we have made important decisions without giving it as much thought as it required. In the end we regretted the outcome or outcomes of our decision.

Indeed, I felt total disappointment with myself for missing out on such an opportunity to shine. I did not take time to think seriously about how participating in the event would benefit my Charity and those around me, especially, my community. I hope I learnt my lesson.

CHAPTER SEVEN
FAITH ACCOMPLISHES THE IMPOSSIBLE

Our Christian life hangs on faith. No one has seen God. It is by faith that we believe that He is, and that He is a Rewarder of those who diligently seek Him (Hebrews 11: 6). If we fail to act in faith, we will never know what it is to trust God; we will always want to do things using human wisdom and reasoning.

When I was nominated as a Torch Bearer, I did not know what it entailed. All that was required was for me to step out in faith, and believe that God can help me to do it. But the point is that I was ignorant about what the whole parade was about. I thought it was for very important people, top athletes, who were renowned in their fields. Of course if I was a sports enthusiast I would have had a better understanding of the Olympics and what it entailed; but I wasn't.

Sometimes in life, we can be called upon to do certain things, or perform certain tasks which we think are beyond our capabilities. However, if we act in faith, and believe we can do it, then we certainly can. For as the Bible says, 'all things are possible' to those who believe. The Bible is replete with stories of people who took steps of faith (Hebrews 11), that enabled them to overcome obstacles and challenges they encountered in their lives and personal circumstances. Faith and absolute (unwavering) trust in God are what we need if we are to do exploits and achieve our full potentials in life.

Today, the World celebrates a number of heroes, who dared to believe they could achieve what no other person had accomplished. One good example is Sir Roger Bannister, who broke the four minute mile record in Oxford, in 1954. Although he did not win the medal he desired in the 1952 Olympics, that did not stop him from aiming higher. Instead, it made him more determined to achieve much more. His goal was to break the four minute mile record, which he eventually achieved. Whilst there would appear to be a controversy over who first reached the peak of Mount Everest, the point is that some people like Sir Edmund Hillary and Tenzing Norgay did so. They were the first to get to the peak of the world's tallest mountain and to return safely in 1953. Achieving such a feat required a level of faith that was extra-ordinary. Although others who had attempted to go up the mountain never returned, that did not put them off. They persevered and 'conquered' that mountain. Recently too, we have read about the 80-year old man who is preparing to climb Mount Everest. Whether or not he achieves it is anyone's guess, but the truth of the matter is that he has his heart set on accomplishing that goal. Like him, we too can accomplish what people say is impossible because we have faith in God, who is able to enable us do all things, because we believe in Him.

The enemy of faith is fear and also doubt. These two attributes make us doubt our capabilities. Thank God that David was not afraid of the size of Goliath, or his boastings. He knew His God, and believed that faith in His God was all he needed to confront Goliath. It was an opportunity too good to be missed.

Life will present us with opportunities, which will require us to take giant steps of faith. Sadly, such opportunities do not come our way every day; a truth that I have since learnt through my own experience. As the popular saying goes 'if you only do what you've always done, you'll only get what you've always got'. If you want a different outcome, you must be ready to do something different, even if it means attempting the impossible. People are called heroes, not because they accomplished what ordinary people accomplish, but because they do the extra-ordinary. It is the 'extra' that requires us to act in faith in most cases.

I recall that when I started the Charity, Book Aid for Africa, it required me to take giant steps of faith. Although I was confronted with all sorts of challenges, including lack of commitment from people, lack of funds and facilities, and insufficient time to do all that it demanded, nevertheless, my absolute faith and trust in God kept me going. I knew in whom I had believed, and was fully persuaded that when He calls us to do something, He gives us the grace and the enablement to do it. He responds to the level of our faith.

CHAPTER EIGHT
WHAT IS WRONG WITH RECOGNITION?

Hosting the London 2012 Olympic Games in England was a big event, and an opportunity for many athletes to fulfill a lifelong ambition of participating in the Games and winning some medals. One of the highlights of the Games is usually the Torch Relay, culminating in the lighting of the cauldron at the Olympic Games Opening Ceremony. For the London 2012 Olympic Games, the Olympic Flame and Torch Relay started at the ancient Olympic Games in Greece after a short ceremony, and was handed over to officials in England on 18 May 2012, with pomp and pageantry. The Flame was carried by 8,000 Torchbearers during the Olympic Torch Relay between 19 May and 27 July 2012, and travelled for a period of 70 days through 1018 communities across the UK, starting from Land's End, before it was received in London on 21 July 2012. The Torchbearers were inspirational people who had made significant achievements for themselves or for their local community. They were nominated by people who knew them and then selected through a ballot process, by 12 judging panels around the UK, giving them the opportunity to 'shine' and to inspire millions of people watching them, not only in their community, but across globe.

One of the reasons why I was not interested in carrying the Olympic Flame was because I did not want to draw attention to myself neither was I seeking fame or recognition. It is possible that others in my shoes would have jumped at the opportunity to be seen and or recognised on the world stage. However, when I set up the Charity, Book Aid for Africa, my motive was not to seek fame or recognition. I saw a need which I felt strongly compelled to respond to. Moreover, given that I work in academia, I am in a position to help others with books and educational resources. So, it has been my pleasure and privilege to try to make a difference in the educational landscape in Africa.

This is not to suggest that there is something wrong with being recognised for great personal achievements, or for making a difference in the lives of others. As a matter of fact, the Bible is replete with stories of people who were recognised and celebrated for their achievements. A good example is that of David's defeat of Goliath. After this great accomplishment, David was celebrated and paraded across the city, and the women came out across the cities of Israel and sang his praise, saying *'Saul has slain his thousands, and David his ten thousands'* (1Samuel 18: 6-7). Besides, in most of His Parables about the Kingdom of God, Jesus talked about God rewarding people for what they had done. Even the little things we do for people, like giving a cup of cold water, in His name, does not go unnoticed. Matthew 25: 31-40 gives us an insight into God's recognition and reward system. It says

"When the Son of Man comes in His glory, and all the holy angels with Him, then He will sit on the throne of His glory. All the nations will be gathered before Him, and He will separate them one from another, as a shepherd divides his sheep from the goats. And He will set the sheep on His right hand, but the goats on the left. Then the King will say to those on His right hand, 'Come, you blessed of My Father, inherit the kingdom prepared for you from the foundation of the world: for I was hungry and you gave Me food; I was thirsty and you gave Me drink; I was a stranger and you took Me in; I was naked and you clothed Me; I was sick and you visited Me; I was in prison and you came to Me.'

"Then the righteous will answer Him, saying, 'Lord, when did we see You hungry and feed You, or thirsty and give You drink? When did we see You a stranger and take You in, or naked and clothe You? Or when did we see You sick, or in prison, and come to You?' And the King will answer and say to them, 'Assuredly, I say to you, inasmuch as you did it to one of the least of these My brethren, you did it to Me.'

This suggests that it is acceptable and quite normal for people to gain recognition for their accomplishments, whether big or small. Therefore, it was right and proper for my work with Book Aid for Africa (BAFA) to be recognised (as long as I do not ascribe the glory to myself). By not accepting my nomination to carry the flame, I missed an opportunity to inspire others and to promote the work of the Charity.

CHAPTER NINE
THE SHOCKING DISCOVERY

There are a number of sporting events around the globe, such as the World Cup, Wimbledon, The Test Series in Cricket, The Commonwealth Games, and so on. However, it appears that the Olympics is one of the greatest sporting event in history. If I am not mistaken, it is the peak of the career of most athletes. Since my childhood, I have heard about the Olympic Games. Hearing about it does not mean that I know much about it. Often times we dabble into things for which we know little or nothing about. It is true that like me, many of us have heard about the Olympic Games, yet how many of us really know its history? It was as if God was trying to open my eyes when He allowed me to witness something that almost shocked the life out of me.

The Olympic Games, which are held every four years, date back to 776 BC, according to historical records. They were dedicated to the Olympian gods and were staged on the ancient plains of Olympia. They continued for nearly 12 centuries, until Emperor Theodosius abolished them in 394 AD as they were considered reminiscent of paganism. The first Olympic Games were in honour of Zeus.

Seven days before the Olympic Flame arrived in Britain there was a big ceremony in Greece at the first venue of the Olympics. The Torch and Relay were important elements of the cultural festivals surrounding the Olympic Games of Ancient Greece. During the Games, a sacred flame burned continually on the altar of the goddess, Hera. In addition, heralds were summoned to travel throughout Greece to announce the Games, declaring a sacred truce for the duration.

A very precise ritual for the lighting of the Flame is followed at every game. It is lit from the sun's rays in a parabolic mirror in front of the Temple of Hera (Queen of the Olympian gods) in Olympia, in a traditional ceremony among the ruins of the home of the Ancient Games. It is then transported by a torch to the place where the games are held. This is usually after a short relay around Greece. After that the Flame is handed over to the new Host City at another ceremony in the Panathenaiko stadium in Athens. When the Flame gets to the Host Country, it is transferred from one Torchbearer to another, spreading what is regarded as a message of peace, unity and friendship. It ends its journey as the last Torchbearer lights the cauldron at the Olympic Games Opening Ceremony in the Olympic Stadium, marking the official start of the Games. The Flame is extinguished on the final day of the Games, at the Closing Ceremony.

I remember watching the Flame lighting ceremony in Greece from the television in my kitchen, where I was trying to prepare dinner for the family. Fortunately, I was not there on my own; my husband and our youngest son were also in the kitchen with me. We all watched the ceremony with our mouths wide open in disbelief, as we got an insight into what the torch bearing was all about. We saw one of the temple priestesses making incantations to the gods of the sun, including Apollo. Ah! It then dawned on me why my spirit was not connected to the event in the first place, even though I was not aware of the historical connection.

The first commandment in the Bible in Exodus 20:3-4 is *"you shall have no other gods before Me. You shall not make for yourself a carved image – any likeness of anything that is in heaven above, or that is in earth beneath, or that is in the water under the earth; you shall not bow down to them nor serve them. For I, the Lord your God, am a jealous God,..."* As a matter of fact, many Israelites were destroyed because of their disobedience in contravening this commandment, and worshipping idols. God utterly detests any form of recognition of any other gods besides Him. And further He says in Isaiah 45: 5, *"I am the Lord, and there is no other; there is no God besides Me'.*

So, here I was watching a ceremony where incantations were being made to other gods, in the name of Olympics. I told my husband and son who were watching the ceremony with me that there was no way I would have carried that Flame if I had accepted my nomination and then selected to do so. I know that a few Christian friends who heard that I had been nominated to carry the Olympic Torch but had not accepted my nomination could not understand how on earth anyone could have declined such an opportunity. I simply told them they would soon find out why. Whereas I had felt really bad for missing such a once in a lifetime opportunity to carry that Torch, the reason was because I was completely ignorant about its history. I wonder how many Christians really know how this whole Olympics came about. It is not surprising to learn that Emperor Theodosius abolished them in 394 AD.

My experience of watching the Flame lighting ceremony in Greece caused me to go and do some research to find out more about the Olympics. I could see from my enquiry that like everything else, there are diverse views about the Olympics, and whether or not Christians should be involved with it. For me, personally, I know what the word of God says, and that is where I stand – *"you shall have no other gods besides Me"*. And in 2Corinthians 6: 17-18, the Bible says *"come out from among them and be separate, says the Lord … And I will receive you. I will be a Father to you, and you shall be My sons and daughters, says the Lord Almighty"*. Why on earth would I want to identify with idol worship?

As if God was trying to confirm this word in my spirit, He sent Rick Pino who led 'FIRE ON THE ALTAR' at Bethshan Church, House of Prayer in Sunderland that week. He spoke on Sunday morning (20 May 2012) on being a voice (John 1: 23; Revelation 4: 5) to the nation – speaking against traditions and many things done in ignorance.

Interestingly, on the day after the names of those who would carry the Olympic Torch was released (8th November 2011), the Trinity Broadcasting Network (TBN) featured the 93rd birthday greetings for a man who had carried the 'Torch' of the Gospel of Jesus Christ across the globe, the right Reverend Billy Graham. Like Rick Pino suggested, Billy Graham has been God's voice across all the continents and carried the Light of the Gospel across the globe. Whilst I was watching the programme, the Holy Spirit spoke very strongly to my heart telling me that it is not about carrying a physical torch, but much more important was carrying the light of the gospel across the world. And, as if to confirm what I had received in my spirit, some of the friends who had read my email in which I had lamented about missing the opportunity to carry the Olympic Torch responded to my email, encouraging me. One of them said *"God will work this out for His glory. He is God after all and you are HIS daughter!"*

Another said *"May God perfect that which concerns you. As you die daily, God will give you beauty for ashes and make His name to be glorified through you. Thank God for your zeal for Him"*.

My brother who had nominated me wrote *"my dearest sister, what else can I say, after I read all you had to say about my nominating you as an Olympics Torch Bearer. You've said it all. I neither can add nor remove an iota of punctuation or word from all that you've said. I however, want you to know how very proud I'm of you and all of your achievements. The hymn writer wrote '... God is His own interpreter ...'. He knows the beginning to the end. That's why He is Alpha and Omega. God's ways are not our ways. He knows best. You are very much appreciated and I know that you always heed the Great Commission of 'go ye into the world and preach my word' at every opportunity. If God really wanted you to bear that Olympics Torch, like Jonah, you wouldn't have had a hiding place. I really didn't realize that I stood the chance of winning a pair of tickets, the compelling force was to nominate a deserving person and to proudly write to Lloyds TSB, about your contributions both spiritually, intellectually and materially to your community and the African continent. Please no more self bashing and continue to serve the Lord, as you've always done ..."*.

Another friend wrote *"what an awesome story ...as I was carefully reading every word you expressed here I could feel your heart of disappointment at yourself for not taking the necessary steps to pursue the torch bearer further ... however most definitely our loving Father already knew that this situation would turn out like this. He knows your heart and that is one of total submission, surrender and servanthood. Many more kairos and serendipitous moments await you. God knows and sees and He has a way of causing all things even the missed opportunities and the disappointments to work together for our good and for His glory. Rejoice in the fact that the Lord knoweth the way that you should go.*

I am also reminded that YOU INDEED DO CARRY THE TORCH ON A DAILY BASIS IN YOUR WALK WITH CHRIST, with those you minister to, with lives you touch through prayer, your daily devotions, your published books, speaking engagements --- YOU ARE ALREADY A TORCH BEARER FOR CHRIST in more ways than one. While it may have been an awesome opportunity to

*participate in such an honorable event ... God is using you to touch
many lives and be a light in dark places in so many ways that you
can't imagine and that impact lives on and on for eternity. KEEP
YOUR TORCH BURNING BRIGHT FOR JESUS!'*

To say that I was greatly encouraged by these replies is an
understatement. As a matter of fact, it appeared that the friend who
wrote the last email, which I reproduced, was reading what the Lord
had laid on my heart.

Given how long I have been on this journey with God, I know He
never lets things happen to me without a purpose. He spoke clearly
to me through the experience to write a book about what it is to be
His Torch Bearer. This last email reply leads us nicely to the other
side of this story!

PART TWO

THE OTHER SIDE OF THE STORY

CHAPTER TEN

An Unforgettable Day

There are certain events that occur in our lives, which are unforgettable. The discovery that I made on the 9th of October 2012 opened up another chapter in my life. I recall that the BBC Reporter, Sarah Hathaway, had described my life as 'dramatic and eventful'. However, after all the 'drama' that have been a reflection of my life, little did I realise that another major drama was going to unfold.

For many of us who travel regularly by plane, we sometimes do not pay attention to flight attendants when they go through their usual safety drills in which they inform passengers about what to do in an emergency. This is because we have heard it so many times over, that we always feel it is a routine exercise and nothing will happen when we are on board a plane. Recently when I heard about a plane that landed on water, I tried to imagine how the passengers would have reacted. They would have had to put into practice the drills that they probably never paid much attention to. Similarly, that is what happens when we attend some talks or seminars where we are taught some things about caring for our bodies, and doing some regular checks on ourselves. We sometimes never take these things seriously until we are faced with the reality. I recall attending a women's conference in 2009 in which we were reminded about the need to examine our breasts regularly, and taught how to do so. Now and again I did try to carry out this check, but I would not say categorically that I have done it every day. However, I recall lying in bed on the morning of Tuesday, 9 October 2012, and I felt an urge to examine my breasts. I examined the left one and it appeared to be fine. But when I examined the right one, I had a very strange feeling. A sudden panic came all over me, as I tried to figure out whether what I was feeling was real or imaginary. What does a lump in your breast feel like? I was not very sure.

In order to make assurance doubly sure, since my GP was a male, I thought that the female nurse in his surgery might be in a better position to tell me whether what I felt on my breast was a real lump or something else. When I tried to make an appointment at my

GP's surgery to see the nurse, I was told she had no free slots until Friday, 12th October. I told myself that there was no way I would wait until Friday with this strange thing in my body. When I told the Receptionist at the surgery that I needed to see the nurse urgently, she then asked what it was I needed to see the nurse about. I told her that I had felt a lump in my breast and that I needed to have it examined to be sure what it was. The receptionist then told me that it was the GP himself that I needed to see and not the nurse. Unfortunately I could not see the GP earlier than Friday. So she made an appointment for me to see my GP on Friday, 12th October at 3.10pm.

It will be impossible for me to quantify the emotions I felt as I was thinking about what was happening. I know that quite a few women die from breast cancer, including some that were personally known to me. Up till this time, I had never heard of any member of my immediate or extended family who had suffered from breast cancer. So, where did this strange thing come from, and why me? These were the thoughts going through my mind. What if the doctor said it was a real lump? Would it be life-threatening? I knew this was going to be a real spiritual battle, if it turned out to be so. Was I mentally, emotionally and physically prepared for what this was going to demand of me? After spending some time in prayer, I went about my business as usual, looking forward to the appointment with my GP, to try and unravel the 'mystery'. Besides my husband and children, I am not sure I mentioned it to anyone else.

On Friday 12th October, I went to see my GP as scheduled. He was a Christian and someone well-known to the family. The Practice Manager was in the room with him when he examined me. He looked at me with mixed emotions and a deep sense of compassion and told me that it was a real lump. In other words, this is no imagination; it is real! Of course I was speechless. I felt tears dropping down my cheeks. He gave me some tissues to dry up my tears and said 'it is well!', and that he hoped the lump would be benign. He then asked me to go and see the Practice nurse who would try to secure an appointment for me to see the Consultant at the Sunderland Royal Hospital (SRH) within two weeks. I met the Practice nurse who told me she could understand how I felt, as she had been in the same situation some sixteen years ago. Fortunately the lump in her breast was benign and she's not had any problems since then. She also tried to encourage me, saying she hoped it would be benign, and that there would be nothing to worry about. I got an appointment to see the Consultant on Monday, 22nd October.

When I got home, I told my husband what had transpired. We prayed and committed everything to God. Until proper tests were carried out, there was nothing to worry about, as we had no idea whether or not the lump was benign or malignant. Life continued as normal, as far as I was concerned. However, I felt anger inside of me that the devil could be so daring. I told myself that he had picked on the wrong person.

Interestingly, my husband and I travelled to London that very day, shortly after seeing my GP. We had a mega engagement in London that weekend, as our friends were having a 3-in-1 celebration, including thanksgiving for complete healing from pancreatic cancer. Yet here I was waiting to find out the nature of the lump in my breast. Nevertheless, the news we heard did not detract nor dampen our spirits. The trip would go on, as planned. As a matter of fact, we stopped at Luton, enroute London, and shared fellowship with close family friends. We also visited two other families in London that weekend. Nobody knew I was facing a personal challenge. And in spite of that challenge, God was using me to bless others. We had a wonderful time in London, to the glory of God.

Besides the trip to London, we were also planning the 5th Anniversary celebration of Book Aid for Africa, on the 27th of October and holding regular meetings. This was a very busy time in my life, and in spite of what was happening to me personally, my spirit was not dampened at all. Although I chaired most of the meetings, there was nothing on my face or my disposition to suggest that I was going through a personal challenge. Whenever I heard some people making excuses at some of our planning meetings about what they could not do, I simply smiled, and thought within me, that if only they knew what was happening to me at this point in time, all those excuses would fade into insignificance. "What kind of 'news' would I hear on the 22nd when I go for my appointment?" I thought. That did not matter; I just got on with life as normal. I have always felt so secure in the love and the faithfulness of God that I knew that He would never take me to any place where His grace will not be sufficient for me.

CHAPTER ELEVEN
THE 'JOURNEY' BEGINS

When I received my appointment letter to see a Consultant at the Sunderland Royal Hospital on the 22nd of October 2012, I was delighted to find out that the Consultant that I had been referred to was someone that I knew personally. So that was reassuring. Interestingly, I had gone to work as usual, and my husband met me there and accompanied me to the hospital. We met with the Consultant, who examined me and asked me to do a mammogram and a scan. He said they needed to ascertain what type of lump was in my right breast. I did all the necessary tests and was asked to return two days later for the result of the tests.

However, as I lay down on the couch watching the radiographer as she was doing the test to ascertain the nature of the lump in my breast, I could not but wonder at what was going on in my body. The picture I saw on the screen was not funny at all. They took a specimen of the lump for further tests and asked me to return two days later for the results of the tests. I was pleasantly surprised when we returned two days later, on the 24th of October 2012, to receive the results of the tests and we were told that the lump was not cancerous. Of course we were very delighted at the news. That is the kind of news most people would want to receive after such a diagnosis. Nevertheless, the Consultant said the lump had to be removed. He also added that the Consultant Histopathologist who carried out the test on the specimen of the lump removed from my breast did say that the kind of substance that was removed from my breast was rare, and that she had never seen such before. Hence the Consultant indicated that the removal of the lump needed to be done urgently so that further tests on it could be carried out to ascertain what kind of substance the tumor contained. I was then scheduled for surgery on the 6th of November.

I was still feeling sore on my right breast because the test that was carried out two days earlier was under local anesthesia. Whilst this 'drama' was unfolding in my life, the 5th anniversary celebration of Book Aid for Africa was scheduled to take place on the 27th of

October. I carried on with my life as normal – intertwining hospital visits with making plans for the anniversary celebration. To the glory of God, the event was successful; no one knew the personal challenge I was facing. Indeed, we can do all things through Christ who strengthens us.

I had important appointments in the South during the weekend of 2nd November to 4th November 2012, meeting with the High Commissioner for Mozambique in London on the 2nd of November, and examining a PhD thesis in Bournemouth on the 5th of November. Yet, I was scheduled for surgery on the 6th of November. How would that be possible? There was no way I could return from a hectic trip one day, and go for surgery the next day. I needed to get my home in order as well as get myself mentally prepared for the challenge ahead. More importantly, I had not had enough time to pray! I told myself that there was no way I would go for surgery on the 6th of November. I rang the hospital just before I travelled to London to let them know I could not come for the surgery on the 6th of November. The Personal Assistant to the Consultant was surprised because she knew the Consultant was keen for me to have the lump removed sooner rather than later.

After I got back from my trip, it was time to do 'business' with my Father, to find out exactly what was going on. I had to set aside some time to fast and pray. It was time for not only some serious dialogue with my Father, but it was also a time for self-examination. Had I done anything wrong, which was why I was going through this? My mother, grandmother, great-grandmother and other females down my family line never had breast cancer. Where on earth did this come from? I needed to hear God speak to me clearly about what was going on. I needed my Rhema word. So I went into the word of God and He spoke to me through a number of scriptures. In John 11:4, He assured me that *'this sickness will not end in death. No, it is for God's glory so that God's Son may be glorified through it'* (NIV). Also in Luke 21: 13, He told me that *'it will turn out as a testimony'* for me. Wow! I was excited. Besides, I digested and regurgitated Psalm 118. Some verses of that chapter came alive in my spirit

'The voice of rejoicing and salvation
Is in the tents of the righteous;
The right hand of the LORD DOES VALIANTLY.

The right hand of the LORD IS EXALTED;
The right hand of the LORD DOES VALIANTLY.
I shall not die, but live,
And declare the works of the LORD.
The LORD HAS CHASTENED ME SEVERELY,
But He has not given me over to death.
Open to me the gates of righteousness;
I will go through them,
And I will praise the LORD.
This is the gate of the LORD,
Through which the righteous shall enter.
I will praise You,
For You have answered me,
And have become my salvation.
(Psalm 188: 15-21, NKJV).

What more did I require when God had given me such reassuring promises?

Besides seeking God's face in prayer and fasting, I embarked on Holy Communion EVERYDAY. Whatever benefits and privileges that I enjoyed as a child of God, it was all through the sacrifice of Christ on the cross for me. So I needed to remind myself of that, and to appropriate those benefits.

Prior to all these developments, Psalm 91 was a Psalm that I prayed DAILY. As a matter of fact, whenever I got to verse 10 that says *'no evil shall befall you, nor shall any plague come near your dwelling'*, I usually spent some time there. So, does it mean that God did not hear my prayers, when verse 15 of the same Psalm says *'he shall call upon Me, and I will answer him; I will be with him in trouble; I will deliver him and honor him?* Of course I know God hears when I call on Him. And I know His love for me is total and complete. Whatever was going on in my life was a temporary challenge.

God's word is a *'lamp unto our feet, and a light to lighten our path'* (Psalm 119: 105). I had to draw a lot of strength from His word during this trying time. One of the stories that encouraged me as I was reflecting on my personal challenge was the story of Job. Here was a man described as *'blameless and upright, and one who feared God and shunned evil'* (Job 1: 1, NKJV). Yet, God allowed him to be tested, because he wanted to showcase him before the devil. Here was I lamenting for missing a once in a life time opportunity to carry an Olympic Torch, yet God had His own idea of torch bearing. How do you bear His torch and let your light shine in a situation such as that in which I found myself? He was already proving Himself faithful in my life up to this point. I was going about my life as normal, in spite of what I was going through, and what was ahead of me.

The Consultant was not happy that I had missed my surgery on the 6th of November. We met with him again on the 9th of November and he still insisted that I needed to have the surgery. I did struggle with this quite a bit. I struggled with the thought of going through surgery in the first place. Why could I not believe that God could heal me and I would not have to go through surgery? Could I not believe that God could make the lump disappear? Interestingly too, the Consultant himself was a Christian, just like my GP. God had chosen to place me in the hands of His children, whom He knew could take care of me.

I believe in healing, and I believe in miracles. I have laid hands on people and Jesus healed them. There have been many times that I prayed for myself and got healed. So why could I not believe that God could remove the lump? Well, like Jesus in the Garden of Gethsemane, facing the daunting prospect of going to the cross, I wrestled with God, until I came to the place of TOTAL and complete SURRENDER, where I said 'Lord, if this cup will not pass from me except I drink it, let Your will be done'.

After we met the Consultant on the 9th of November, he arranged for me to have my lump removed on the 20th of November. He was scheduled to go on a two-week holiday, and wanted to do the surgery before his holiday. So the surgery was booked for 20th November. However, between the 9th and 20th of November, there were quite a few events and activities taking place around me, which I attended, yet there was no indication that I was going through this challenge. Through God's grace on my life, I went about my normal duties in spite of it all.

Before I went for the surgery on the 20th of November, I mentioned it to my Line Manager, being our new Associate Dean. Fortunately, he did not ask me what kind of surgery it was. But it was important that he knew I would be away from work for a few days. The Consultant had mentioned that many women reacted differently to the treatment. Some returned to work immediately, whilst others stayed home for a few days. I was not sure what would happen in my own case.

On Sunday, 18th of November, after the worship service at Newcastle, I informed our Pastor that I was going in for surgery on Tuesday, and he prayed with me and my husband. I also mentioned it to another couple in the church, and that was it. My husband accompanied me to the hospital on the day of the surgery. It was a day case, and I was home later in the evening to the glory of God.

CHAPTER TWELVE

'ARE YOU ON YOUR OWN'?

After my excisional surgery on the 20th of November, I returned to Sunderland Royal Hospital (SRH) on the 28th of November for my post-op review, and to have part of my stitches removed. I met with my Consultant Surgeon who mentioned that the Histopathologist at SRH had said she had never seen the type of lump removed from my breast before. The multi-disciplinary team (MDT) had met and was discussing the best way forward with my case. In the mean time, they had decided to send the specimen taken from the lump in my breast to the Regional Consultant Histopathologist at the Queen Elizabeth Hospital in Gateshead. I found that really interesting. I kept on wondering at what was this drama that was unfolding before my very eyes? Imagine how you would feel if you were in my shoes and heard something like that. All I kept on saying to myself was that 'God was going to get the glory out of this; the devil is a LIAR!'

The Consultant Surgeon had mentioned that he would be away on holiday the following week, but I had actually forgotten about that when I returned to SRH for my next appointment on the 6th of December. This time it was a different doctor that I met, and he was with a Macmillan nurse. It so happened that in addition to sending the specimen from my lump to the Regional Histopathologist, they had also sent it to the National Histopatologist. However, due to work commitments, my husband could not accompany me on this visit, so I was on my own (with King Jesus, of course). The doctor asked me if there was anyone with me, I replied 'no', but in my heart I knew I was not on my own. He then told me that they were still waiting for the result from the National Pathologist, but that the Regional Pathologist said the test results showed a rare form of depressed cancer. Wow!!! Where did that come from? The devil is a LIAR!!! How would you feel if after you had been told that the lump they found in your breast was benign, and now to hear this type of news? This was why the doctor had asked if I was on my own. He was going to give me the type of news that would require someone to be there with me. I took a deep breath and whispered a prayer. I felt a lump in my throat. I wanted to cry but did not know how. The doctor left the room, and I was with the Macmillan nurse. You could see compassion written all over her face. Indeed, she understood what it is like to receive such news. That is what she has been trained for, to look after people who receive such news and to be there for them. Now I was embarking on a journey that nothing had prepared me for. (Now I'm really trying to hold back my tears as I write this. The memory is too painful). But I was determined not to let anything rob me of my joy. I knew that I was secure in the love of God and that if he had allowed this it was that His name will be glorified. Special trials are reserved for special people. If God preserved me in the womb of my mother when I was helpless and could not defend myself, would He abandon me now? Not really!

The interesting thing of course was that in spite of my surgery, I was back to work as normal, even before I went for this appointment. The only thing I could not do was driving the car myself because of the pain on my right breast. But on this occasion I drove to the hospital myself. People at work had no clue what was happening with me. They saw me come in and out of work as I always did, and I carried on with my duties as normal.

Now alone with the Macmillan nurse, she asked about the general state of my health, my age etc. When I told her my age she said I did not look my age at all, for which I thanked her. And I thanked God, too, for He is the One who renews my youth as the eagle. The nurse told me that I would have to do some blood tests and that I would have to come in the following week for a CT scan. She said she would love to bring me in much earlier, if possible. She handed me her complimentary card, as well as a pack containing information about the treatment of breast cancer. I gave her my mobile phone number in case she needed to contact me to rearrange any of my appointments. She removed the rest of my stitches that day, and then I went on to have my blood samples taken. However, before she left, I told the nurse that there was no room for cancer in my body, and that the devil was only wasting his time.

Interestingly, in spite of the news I had received, the tests and so on, I returned to the University and got back to work as normal. I suppose the devil got what he deserved, a slap on the face. If he thought my world would crumble on hearing such news, he chose the wrong person. We can, and we will always do 'all things through Christ' who strengthens us.

The next day, out of the blues, as it were, I received a strange text message from one of the young ladies that I mentor. She was asking about my general welfare and said she saw my enemy (not me!) in her dream and the person was seriously ill. I told her that when she has such dreams she should pray and cancel it. She told me she did. I was quite taken aback by this dream, but not surprised, knowing that the devil never means well for God's children. I spent most of that day waiting on God, and anointed my whole body with anointing oil, and had Holy Communion.

My husband and I were back at the hospital on the 11th of December for my CT scan, which was necessary to examine my ovaries, pancreas and appendix. We went back the next day to see the Consultant Surgeon for the results of the tests as well as find out if they had heard from the National Histopathologist. This time the wait was long. The multi-disciplinary meeting went on for much longer than normal (over one and half hours). As we sat in the waiting area, I was wondering whether all that discussion was about me, or were there other cases being considered as well?

When we eventually met with the Surgeon, he told us that they had now heard from the National Histopathologist, and that she confirmed that the substance they found in the lump in my breast was rare, and that only four of such cases had been recorded in medical literature. He said the MDT decided that a wider local excision around the area of the breast that was opened up would be necessary, and that he would also do the removal of one of the nodes in my armpit. This was scheduled to take place on Saturday, 15th of December at 8.00am. I was asked to go and do a sentinel node biopsy the next day.

Wait a minute! What does it mean to have a rare form of cancer, and why me? Well, why should I ask that question, knowing how really special I know I am to God? If he chooses me to bear His Torch, and to shine His light, how could I expect that I would have what every other person has? I thought I had made enough medical history in the womb of my mother when I survived abortion. I had survived death, abduction, and other extreme circumstances. Now I'm also making medical history? How interesting is that?

Surprisingly, a few weeks after this appointment with the Surgeon, I received a letter from one of the surgical trainees at SRH who was part of the Breast Surgery team. He said that he was writing to me about my recent breast surgery because 'the nature of the lump that was removed is very rare' and that he would like my permission 'to write up the case for submission to a medical journal for publication'. He enclosed a copy of the proposed report, including some pictures of the lump. I thought 'hm! this is getting really interesting'. I was wondering what exactly was going on? Where is this leading? What can I say, of course, I gave him the permission to do so. If I am in the World to be God's Torch Bearer, what else would I expect? If through my pain other lives can be saved, so be it.

In everyday parlance, we all know what it is like, to 'open up old wounds'. These are certain issues or areas in our lives that are like 'tipping points'. They are sore areas, representing past events or happenings that we do not want to be reminded of. I have a few of those myself, like my experience in Exeter in 1995, when I came face to face with man's inhumanity to man. For some people it might be mentioning an ex-wife, ex-husband, or the loss of a loved one. Nobody likes to have old wounds opened up. So, when the Surgeon told me he would have to go back to the spot where I had my first surgery and open it up again, I thought, 'this guy must be joking'. How on earth is that going to happen? Now I knew I was in for something really serious. The prospect of that surgery was quite daunting. When we got home that evening, my husband rang up another doctor friend of ours, and he came to the house to see us. We told him what was happening, and he tried to explain why these additional measures were being taken. It was an extreme measure to ensure there would be no re-occurrence of the lump.

CHAPTER THIRTEEN

LIFE AT THE WARD

I was back at the SRH on the 14th of December for my sentinel node biopsy. This was necessary to help identify the lymph nodes under my armpit that will be removed, and to know if the deadly disease had travelled to other parts of my body. Wow! That was another drama. This experience has opened my eyes to a whole new world of medical science, and to see how much it has advanced. I even had a little chat with the lady (medical physicist) who carried out the biopsy to find out where she had studied, and she confirmed she had studied at Sunderland University. I was quite impressed with her professionalism and the sophistication of the equipments that she used.

15th of November was not a day I was looking forward to at all. Nevertheless, I had committed myself and all that was happening, to God. My life was in His hands. Whereas the surgery on the 20th of November was a day case, this second surgery was to take place in ward D47. I did mention it to my Associate Dean that I was going in for another surgery, but again he did not ask what it was about, which was great. So, again, I was saved from having to tell stories. The point is that I did not like to talk about what was happening in my life at this time because I was not ready to glorify sickness, or to let the devil think he got the upper hand. No he didn't, because my life continued as fairly normal as possible.

My husband dropped me off at the SRH very early on the morning of 15th December. I went to ward D47 and sat in the waiting area, not knowing what I was expected to do. I sat there until one of the ladies came and took me to the ward and showed me my bed. I noticed that they whisked one lady to the theatre, and after that they came for me. I had the wider local excision as well as the removal of one of the nodes under my armpit.

This time, the experience was much different from the first one. I had two surgeries in one go, and I did not feel well at all. When I was taken back to the ward, God opened my eyes to see what women like me were going through. I was in the ward with women whose conditions appeared worse than mine. One of them actually had a mastectomy; another had tubes all over her as her blood was being drained. The most heart-breaking for me was the young lady on the opposite side of my bed, who groaned all through the night. Her jaw had been damaged when a tube was being passed through her throat and she was in indescribable pain. I knew God had placed me in the ward for a purpose, but at that point in time, all I needed was sleep. I was feeling very dizzy and faintish, and could hardly open my eyes. Even when my husband and another sister, who was a consultant at the hospital, visited me at the ward, I barely knew what was happening around me.

Now my surgery had taken place in the morning hours. By the time I was taken to the ward, it was nearing the visiting hours from 2.00pm. The lady next to me had lots of people visiting her. This meant every effort I made to catch some sleep was useless. After the visitors left at 5pm, it was time for supper, and shortly after that it would be the next visiting time. I found myself asking why I had private health insurance if I was languishing away in this type of place, where I was not even guaranteed a decent sleep. I was feeling very exhausted. After the visiting time for the day was over, I heaved a sigh of relief and thought I could eventually lie down and have some rest. That was wishful thinking.

After their visitors left, these two ladies in the ward could not stop talking. My, oh my! I was desperate; I wanted to cry, but was even too weak to do so. I knew I was being kept in the ward so that I could recover fully from the effect of the anesthesia, yet here I was not able to get the sleep I desperately needed. At some point, I felt like asking my husband to come and take me home. As a matter of fact, when I was able to manage to walk on my own, without support, I went over to the nurses and asked if they had a spare room somewhere where I could sleep. It was getting to nearly 10pm at night, and I was still trying to get some sleep. The nurses looked at me as if I came from another world. One of them calmed herself down and said they would shortly be turning the lights off, and that they had no spare room or bed anywhere. They appeared quite hostile. However, as I overhead the conversation between these two women, I understood why God wanted me to remain in the ward that night. I told my husband not to bother coming to take me home, instead when he was coming to see me the next day, he should come with some of my books, as I had some business to do with these women. When I could not take it any longer, I told the ladies that I had been trying to get some sleep all day, without much success. I was not being anti-social, but I really needed to sleep. I told them that when I got up in the morning, we would have the opportunity to have a real chat, because I found the subject of their discussion quite interesting.

When I eventually fell asleep, in the middle of the night, I heard the lady opposite me groaning all through the night. I think her pain was too overwhelming for her. It made my heart ache so badly. I felt quite helpless, as I was too weak and tired to do anything. I simply prayed for her on my bed. In the morning, my husband came to see me and brought copies of my books, which I freely distributed to the ladies in the ward. I shared the gospel with the two who had been chatting together the previous day. I noticed that a young girl, about the age of 16 or 17years arrived and occupied the bed next to mine. I did not know what procedure she came for, but when the lady next to her bed on the other side told me what it was, my spirit groaned within me. I also gave her a copy of my book, but I noticed she was not on her bed when I was leaving. That made me sad, as I did not have the opportunity to share with her. However, I went over quietly to the bed of the young lady opposite me, who had groaned all night, and asked if I could pray for her. She consented, and I did. In a way, I was grateful to God for the opportunity I had to share the love of God with these ladies. I believe the fruit of that encounter will remain throughout eternity.

CHAPTER FOURTEEN
HUG IN A BAG?

After my discharge from the hospital, a few friends visited us at home. Some brought me food, for which I shall ever remain grateful. I went for my post-op assessment on the 20th of December, and met the surgeon and the nurse. I was informed that the result of the nymph node removal was not yet available. Also the MDT had not met, so it was not yet clear what treatment plan I would require.

I had taken little Christmas presents and thank you cards with me for this appointment to give to the Consultant Surgeon and the nurse. In return, the nurse handed me a gift bag, which had the inscription '**HUG in a bag**'. This created some curiosity in me, and I was keen to see the contents of the bag. In addition to the bag, she gave me a heart-shaped cushion to place under my arm to enable lie down comfortably in bed because I had told her that I was having difficulty placing my right arm close to my side.

When I got home and brought out the things in the bag, I opened my mouth wide in amazement. I could not believe my eyes. The bag was full of all sorts of goodies for women going through breast cancer treatment. There were some leaflets and a card in the gift bag, which explained the idea behind the concept of 'HUG in a Bag'.

HUG, stands for **Help** (a useful list of contacts), **Understanding** (from women who have undergone the same experiences) and **Glamour** (a selection of beauty products). I was deeply moved. This for me, is what life is about – making a difference in the lives of others, through our own experiences. Whilst some people moan and groan about what they have been through, others see their experience as an opportunity to help others who would face similar situations – make the 'load' much lighter for them when they have to go through the same experience. The card in the bag had the title 'A HUG for You!', and read.

*It's amazing what
a hug can do –
a hug can cheer you
when you're blue,
a hug can soothe
the hurt and pain
and bring a rainbow
after rain...*

*A hug can say
"you're doing fine"
Or, "you'll be better
In no time"
The hug – there is
No doubt about it ...
we never could
survive without it!*

*So here's a hug
Without delay
Just to cheer you up
Today!*

Love Hugo
X

HUG in a Bag is a non-profit organization 'formed by three women who met, laughed, cried and supported each other during their treatment for breast cancer. Each of the three coped in their own way but found that sharing their thoughts, anxieties and concerns was extremely helpful. They also gave each other lots of hugs in times of fear, sadness and joy!' The aim of these women is to give 'one more hug in the form of a bag containing gifts, information leaflets and discount vouchers to every person diagnosed with breast cancer in Sunderland Royal Hospital'. This is because they know from their own experience that women can feel very alone and vulnerable at this time, and they wanted to show their understanding and support.

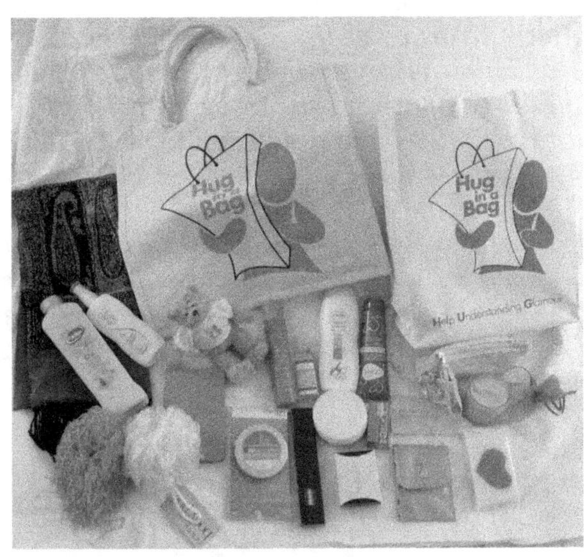

The action of these three women reminds me of a Cable News Network (CNN) programme (*CNN Heroes*) that my husband and I stumbled on to recently. The programme was essentially about people who understood how to turn their trials into triumphs; their pain, into other people's gain. I was particularly touched by the story of the little 12 year old Jessie Rees, who during her 10 month courageous fight with two brain tumours created 'JOYJARS', which were used to spread hope, joy and love to children fighting life altering medical illnesses across America in homes and hospitals. Each JOYJAR holds 15-20 new, age-appropriate toys. She came up with the four letter words, NEGU, that are now synonymous with the foundation, created after she lost her battle with cancer. NEGU stands for Never Ever Give Up. How awesome is that?

In Philippians 1: 12-14, the Apostle Paul said *I want you to know, brothers, that what has happened to me has really served to advance the gospel, so that it has become known throughout the whole imperial guard and to all the rest that my imprisonment is for Christ. And most of the brothers, having become confident in the Lord by my imprisonment, are much more bold to speak the word without fear"*.

This is what the Lord wants us to do regarding the trials of life that confront us, to use them as a means for the furtherance of the gospel as well as to make a difference in the lives of others. In 2Corinthians 4: 17-18, Apostle Paul says *"for this light momentary affliction is preparing for us an eternal weight of glory beyond all comparison, as we look not to the things that are seen but to the things that are unseen. For the things that are seen are transient, but the things that are unseen are eternal"*.

When we are facing or have gone through a life- changing encounter, our attitude should be 'Lord, how can I use this experience to help others? No one should go through what I've been through, and even if they have to go through it, I want to use my experience to help them get through it triumphantly'.

CHAPTER FIFTEEN

SUDDENLY!

Like the previous couple of years, my family had decided that I would not do any cooking for Christmas. They did not want me to strain myself at all, following my surgery. In addition, a Christian family in obedience to the Lord, also brought us a very large-size roast turkey. This was to ensure that I did not have to prepare the turkey, either. I was absolutely overwhelmed with the gestures of kindness I received during this period. My younger brother and his family visited us during the Christmas season and we all had a lovely time together. My special caterer daughter in the Lord that God blessed us with did not disappoint at all with her array of spread for our Christmas meal. She exceeded all expectations, and it has never ceased to amaze me where she gets her energy from.

Generally I felt well and strong, and did not show signs of someone who was recovering from surgery. I still managed to organise Christmas presents for family and friends, although because of the surgeries on my breast and on my lymph nodes, I could not drive for some time. However, I was given a leaflet at the hospital of regular exercises I needed to do to ensure I maintained movement in my right arm.

The MDT at SRH had still not met when I went for my next appointment on the 28th of December, according to the Consultant Surgeon, who I met with the nurse. However, the stitches on my lymph nodes and alternate stitches on my right breast were removed. I was given another appointment to come to the hospital on the 2nd of January 2013.

On the last Saturday of the year, the 29th of December, I was delighted that I could still take part in the Kids' Club that we run in Washington, although of course I could not participate in any vigorous activity. On the last Sunday of the year in church, I made the devil truly sorry, with the radical praise I gave to God on that day. If he thought he could rob me of my joy with all that was happening in my life, he was wasting his time.

I recall that when I was preparing for the second round of surgery, the Consultant had mentioned that one of the risks of the wider local excision was the risk of infection. So, before I went for the surgery, and even on the day of the surgery, my husband and son left no stones unturned at home, as they tried to clean everywhere.

The end of year service on the 31st of December has always been one that I looked forward to. This particular one would not be an exception. However, on the morning of the 31st of December, as I went into the kitchen to have something to eat, I noticed that my cooking hob needed a bit of cleaning. So I decided to give it a little scrub, using my right hand, of course. After all, I had been instructed to exercise that hand.

After our dinner that evening, I felt quite a bit of pain under my arm and on my right side generally, and was also very tired. So I decided that I would take a nap before the All Night Prayer Meeting to usher in the New Year. I chose to lie down on the 3-seater sofa in our lounge so that I would not sleep past the time we would need to be at the church. But as I was trying to sleep, I felt very unwell and dizzy, and the pain intensified. I took some pain killers and staggered upstairs and jumped into bed. I told my husband that I could not go anywhere with the way I was feeling. I suggested he could go and that I would be fine. He said there was no way he would leave me feeling unwell and go for the All Night Prayer meeting. So we were both at home.

I woke up on the morning of the New Year and felt like I was actually dying. I could not even move myself in bed. That was how bad the pain on my breast was. I could not eat either. I felt feverish and completely helpless. Prior to this time, life was fairly normal. Not many people knew what I was going through, not even at work or at the Church. Fortunately the second surgery took place close to the Christmas break, so I had no reason to be off sick from work. However, what I was facing at this point in time was different.

Thank God He saw me through the first day of the year. We were still able to wish friends and family a 'happy New Year', although much later in the evening. I went to bed that night and then suddenly, something happened. I saw myself dripping with some dirty looking fluid from my right breast. My clothes were wet and the bed too. Wow!!! 'What is this?' I exclaimed. Nothing prepared me for this phase in my drama. My right breast was swollen and very painful. When the Consultant talked about the risk of infection following wider local excision, I had no idea what he meant, or what I should expect. Sadly, I did not ask him, either. So, what I encountered on the morning of 2nd January scared the life out of me and my husband.

My husband ran downstairs and brought out some plasters and dressings from our First Aid kit. We put them over the dressing that was there to try to stop the dripping. Fortunately, I had an appointment at the SRH that very day, so that was such a welcome relief. We went for the appointment and met the Consultant. It was a different nurse that was there this time. My assigned nurse had mentioned she would be on holiday when I came for my next appointment. The Consultant examined my breast and said there was a build-up of fluid. I was in so much pain as he tried to evacuate the fluid, which was hot and very messy. He said I had a slight infection and prescribed some antibiotics and a stronger pain killer. I was given some dressing for my wound. For the rest of the week, my husband and I had a routine of waking up in the night to dress my wound, which was always dripping.

I was to examine a PhD thesis in Southampton during the first week of January, and another one at Teeside University in the third week. I had to email them to have both rescheduled. My next hospital appointment was scheduled for the 4th of January, and this time my assigned nurse was back. The Consultant tried to squeeze out more pus and to cleanse it. Wow! How painful that was! He prescribed a different type of antibiotic. When I asked if I would have to pay again for another prescription, the nurse gave me an NHS Exemption form to fill so that I would not have to pay for my prescriptions. Does that mean I would be requiring a lot of medication as I went through this drama? 'No', I told myself. I would not need that exemption certificate; the devil is a liar! Whilst reflecting on the infection in my wound, the nurse said she had not seen one so bad. That was a real experience for me, and one that I may never forget. Again, it appeared that everything about my diagnosis and the outcome were unique, confirming again that I was on a special assignment.

The first Saturday of the month was usually when the Overseas Fellowship of Nigerian Christians (OFNC) had their regular meeting. My husband and I were scheduled to lead the first meeting of the year. Unfortunately I was not in a position to attend, so he went alone. The Branch Coordinator and another family came to visit after the meeting. They brought me some food, for which I was very grateful.

My next hospital appointment was on the 9th of January. The last few stitches on my breast were removed, and the procedure was quite painful. The Consultant then said that my treatment would be followed up with radiotherapy. He said it was necessary to follow up such procedures with radiotherapy to ensure that the tumour does not return. 'Radio...what?' I thought within myself. I had heard of radiotherapy, chemotherapy and so on but I never thought it was something I would experience in my life. I felt like saying to the Consultant, 'oh! don't worry, I'll be fine; I don't think I'll need that'. But somehow, I did not do that. Jesus did not stop half way, as much as He was tempted in the Garden of Gethsemane to let the 'cup' pass Him by. I had already come to the place of total surrender on this matter myself, so I would not stop half-way. I told myself that God was free to do with me whatever He desired.

Before we left, I gave the Consultant and the nurse a copy each of my book, *The Greatest Debtor to His Love – and a Trophy of His grace*. I told the nurse that another book would emerge from my experience. She looked at me in amazement and gave me some leaflets to help me understand my radiotherapy treatment and what it would entail.

On Saturday, 12 January 2013, I checked my wound and found it was completely dry. What a relief! I would no longer need to have any dressing on. This meant that I could actually have a real shower without any fear of my wound being wet. Wow!!! What a feeling I had when that happened. These are the little things we take for granted.

My younger sister had visited us the previous week and brought me some fruit juices, including beetroot juice. I use beetroot in my salad regularly but had never drunk it as juice. I think I took a small glass before I left for work on Friday, 18th of January. That evening, I was still at work, and had gone to the toilet and emptied my bowels. As I got up to flush the toilet bowl, I was petrified with what I saw in that bowl. I know I have had near death encounters and experiences that made the BBC Reporter describe my life as 'dramatic and eventful'. The discharge from my breast did scare me, but I don't think that compared with how I felt on this particular evening. When you're undergoing treatment for what is described as a 'rare form of cancer', anything can happen. In fact, you do not know what to expect. The liquid in the toilet bowl was pure red and my stool looked rather strange. I feared the worst. I could not get my eyes off the toilet bowl. I told myself that there was no way I would not get these specimens tested. I called up my husband, who was in the Library at the time working. I told him what had happened and that I needed to go the Accident and Emergency immediately so they could test my stool and the specimen of my urine. Again I felt like death was probably around the corner, and that some of the organs in my body had been badly damaged and that I was bleeding internally. Oh! my God! The feeling was horrible.

I cannot recall how many times and for how long I stared into the toilet bowl. However, as I was walking back to my room, I felt the urge within me to phone my younger sister to ask her a few questions. I asked her what kind of stool and urine one would expel after taking beetroot juice. I told her what had just happened to me. She said she was sorry she had not alerted me of what I should expect after drinking beetroot juice; that your stool and urine will be coloured red, like blood. My God! what a relief I felt. I then rang my husband not to panic that I had confirmed with my sister the reason for the change in my stool and urine. I telephoned my sister and told her it would be better for her to come and collect the rest of the beetroot juice since she was already used to taking it. I did not think it was advisable for me to continue to take it, given the effect it had on me. That experience was overwhelming, and I would not wish for anyone to feel the way I felt that evening.

My last appointment at the SRH before the commencement of my radiotherapy treatment was on the 23rd of January. After examining me, the Consultant said I would be receiving a letter from the Freemans Hospital in Newcastle giving details of my radiotherapy treatment. I would also be receiving a letter from them inviting me for a review of my progress after six months.

CHAPTER SIXTEEN

THIS IS REALITY

On the 24th of January, I received a phone call from one of the staff at Freemans Hospital arranging for me to come in to prepare for my radiotherapy. An appointment was fixed for the 31st of January 2013.

I thought I had enough trouble already, with all the challenges I had faced in the past few months. So when another terrible pain developed on the left side of my neck close to my throat on Monday, 28th January after my marathon teaching session, I was very upset. I kept on asking 'what is this again?' Initially I thought the pain was on my gum and I used Bonjela for two days. I placed my hands on my neck and prayed. I also took some pain killers. I felt some relief, but as I was teaching on Wednesday, 30th of January, the pain was unbearable. I called my dentist to make an appointment thinking it was something to do with my gum. However the time scheduled for the appointment (2.10pm) coincided with the time (2.00pm) I had scheduled to see my PhD students. I was not happy with that arrangement. On second thought, I called my GP's surgery for an emergency appointment. They offered me one at 1.10pm. I thought that was a much better timing and then cancelled the appointment with the dentist. I told them I needed to see my GP first and that if he felt it was a dental problem, then I would come back to them.

I went for my appointment with my GP and we both looked at each other. I could feel tears coming down my cheeks. We both remembered the last time I was there and all that had transpired since that first meeting and the confirmation of the lump in my breast on Friday, 12th October 2012. I had not been back to his surgery since then. He always used the expression 'it is well!' Of course I understood what he meant. I told him that some of us had been chosen by God to showcase His love and to bear His light. He also understood what I meant, having been inundated with letters from the Consultant looking after me at SRH giving him updates on my treatment. He gave me a prescription for antibiotics, and I left his consulting room, determined not to give in to my emotions.

Since most of my classroom teaching was in the second semester, my radiotherapy treatment would affect some of my classes. Prior to this time, only my Associate Dean knew I had gone in for surgery a couple of times. That notwithstanding, I was still in and out of work, as much as possible. It so happened that the worse part of my illness took place during the Christmas break when the University was on holiday. This meant that no one knew what was going on. I was back at work in January like everyone else when the University resumed. Given that one of my teaching sessions would be affected during the radiotherapy treatment, I had to alert the Associate Dean, the Resources Manager and my Team Leader so they would arrange cover for some of my classes.

I recall how shocked my Team Leader was when I told him I was going for post-op treatment at the Freeman Hospital. He said he never knew I had had surgery. Again, no one asked what type of treatment I was going for, so there was no need to tell stories. It is only through the special grace of God that such can happen. I know that some members of my family and even some friends had asked why I did not consider taking time off work, giving what was happening in my life. I know some ladies who went off work for six months once they had the type of diagnosis that I had. I recall telling someone that I was not prepared to glorify sickness in my body. As far as I was concerned, my healing was complete on the cross of Christ, and that the devil was only wasting his time.

On Thursday, 31 January, I went for this 'Treatment Planning' that I had heard so much about. Due to work commitments, my husband could not accompany me on this occasion; instead I got a lift off our first son, who fortunately was off work on that day. I had been reading about radiotherapy to familiarise myself with what to expect. So, there was nothing new that I heard from the Consultant Oncologist that I met at the Newcastle Centre for Cancer Care (NCCC). What was interesting was the comment the Consultant made when she was looking through my notes. She said 'this is the lady whose story has gone all over the country'. She said that even the National Pathologist put an exclamation mark in her comments that she had never seen anything like this before. That is, the lump that was removed from my breast.

Oftentimes, we can be so distant from what goes on in the lives of others until it gets close to home. How often did I receive leaflets through our letter box to support Macmillan Cancer Trust, or Marie Curie Cancer Care, or other charities that are aimed at people suffering from cancer? Did I understand the magnitude of the impact of cancer on the lives of others, until I visited this Centre? Not really. How many precious lives do you know that have been cut short through cancer? It is not easy for anyone to understand the impact that cancer has in the lives of people until it gets close to you. I recall that as we drove past Freeman Hospital, to get to the NCCC, I never knew what to expect. I never knew that such a place existed. It is well worth visiting that place, as it drives reality home. The experience was quite humbling.

My first radiotherapy treatment was on Tuesday 26th of February. The hospital had tried to arrange my treatment around my husband's work schedule as well as those of others who would be giving me lifts to the hospital daily (Monday to Friday) for 3 weeks. One of the side effects of radiotherapy I was told was fatigue. The suggestion was that I should stay off work for three weeks during my treatment. Again, I spent some time in prayer and fasting before I commenced this treatment. I also anointed my whole body with anointing oil for 7 consecutive days. I used no lotion or cream except anointing oil on my body. I told God that this radiotherapy treatment will not harm my body in any way; neither would I suffer any side effects from it. As a matter of fact, I called it 'Fire of the Holy Ghost Therapy'. I knew God heard my prayer.

I had different people taking me for my treatment daily, my husband, first son, second son, and a friend. What amazed me during my daily visits to the NCCC, was the large numbers of people who attend treatment for one form of cancer or the other. I was pleased that two of our sons had the experience of visiting NCCC, so that they would understand what was going on in the lives of others around us. One thing that was intriguing about it all was that you would see these people on the road and they would appear as normal as possible. How many people in my place of work had any idea of what was going on in my life? Not one! Not even the students I was teaching had any idea of what was going on in my life, as I never missed any classes except the two afternoon sessions on a Monday that clashed with my treatment schedule. Things are not always as they appear on the surface.

This reminds me of the day I had my first surgery on the 20th of November 2012. As I sat in the hospital lounge at the SRH waiting for my husband to come and collect me, I picked up one of the magazines (*'Heart Matters'*) on the table that caught my attention. One of the features in the magazine was the experience of a 68 year old lady who was sharing how she was still trying to make the most of her life in spite of her personal circumstances - has had two heart attacks, suffered a divorce, although still close to her ex husband, he died. And worse still, she lost her only son, a 24 year old man who was a deep-sea diver, who never returned from one of his diving expeditions. As a mother of three sons myself, I could not imagine what that must feel like. Usually when you lose a loved one, you can put closure to it by giving them a befitting burial. But what happens when everyday you wake up trying to imagine what must have befallen your most loved, and only child?

As I was thinking about this, my mind also went to the BBC Panorama (I think it was called 'Mind Reader'), which featured some families who were faced with the challenges of caring for their sons who had been involved in accidents that caused damage to their brains. It was difficult for me to try to imagine what such a challenge must feel like - living with someone who was as good as 'dead' and yet still giving them all the love and attention? There was nothing to suggest that any of these families were Christians or believers as we would class them. Yet it was amazing to see what the grace of God could do in their lives.

As we drove home from the hospital, I said to my husband, "people are going through some stuff". I told him about what I read in the magazine and recalled the BBC panorama as well. In my own case, here I was coming out of hospital following a surgery, after having been in and out of hospital for some 4-5 weeks undergoing all sorts of tests and finding the prospect of a surgery rather daunting. Yet I went about my duties as normal, putting the needs of others before mine, and trying to do all I could to get on with life, in spite of what was happening. Not many knew I was facing such a health challenge in my own life. I also knew there were things I wish I could do that I was not able to do, or places and or events I was invited to that I was unable to attend. It is possible that some people would have misjudged me wrongly, because they had no idea of the challenge I was facing. And guess what? The Holy Spirit spoke so strongly to my heart.

The fact is that, every single person we come across is facing a challenge. It could be physical, mental, emotional, financial or otherwise. This is why we must be careful how we jump into conclusions about people, judge or condemn others because we have no clue what they must be going through. This is why my husband would always say 'you must give people the benefit of the doubt'. How we need to pray that the Lord will help us to have a more caring attitude, to be nice to people - a kind word, a smile, etc. We cannot underestimate what these things could mean to people. This is what it is to be a TORCH BEARER, to carry the light of His love with us EVERYDAY. We are to "have the mind of Christ", who was ALWAYS MOVED WITH COMPASSION for people. Rather than judge wrongly, criticise or condemn others, let us whisper a prayer for them and ask God to meet them at their points of need, because you have no clue what is going on in their lives. And we are admonished to *'owe no man nothing, but love'* (Romans 13: 8, NKJV).

How can I forget a personal experience a few years back when I met a ragged middle-aged man who had stumbled into a fellowship meeting looking for help and no one took notice of him; I went gently to him and placed my hands on his shoulders. This man looked straight into my eyes and asked "is there hope for someone like me?" My, oh my! Can I ever forget how much I wept that day and how this man wept also? After I calmed down, I held him closely and told him there was hope for him, and shared God's love with him. To cut the story short, this man (John) prayed and invited Jesus into his life. We gave him a bible, and the immediate transformation of his countenance was visible for all to see.

Isaiah 61: 1-3 reminds us of what would be evident in our lives when the Spirit of the Lord comes upon us, when we become His Torch bearers: He anoints us *"To preach good tidings to the poor; ...to heal the brokenhearted, To proclaim liberty to the captives, And the opening of the prison to those who are bound; To proclaim the acceptable year of the LORD, And the day of vengeance of our God; To comfort all who mourn, To console those who mourn in Zion, To give them beauty for ashes, The oil of joy for mourning,*

The garment of praise for the spirit of heaviness; That they may be called trees of righteousness, The planting of the LORD, that He may be glorified."

Steve Green in his song *'People Need the Lord'* drives this truth home.

.

Every day they pass me by,
I can see it in their eyes.
Empty people filled with care,
Headed who knows where?

On they go through private pain,
Living fear to fear.
Laughter hides their silent cries,
Only Jesus hears.

People need the Lord, people need the Lord.
At the end of broken dreams, He's the open door.
People need the Lord, people need the Lord.
When will we realize, people need the Lord?

We are called to take His light
To a world where wrong seems right.
What could be too great a cost
For sharing Life with one who's lost?

Through His love our hearts can feel
All the grief they bear.
They must hear the Words of Life
Only we can share.

People need the Lord, people need the Lord
At the end of broken dreams, He's the open door.
People need the Lord, people need the Lord.
When will we realize that we must give our lives,
For people need the Lord.

People need the Lord.

We are the embodiment of Christ – His hands, feet, eyes, ears and all! Let us go about our daily activities being His true ambassadors and representing His kingdom and doing what He would have done if He was physically with us today. He has left us an example (of love, humility, selflessness, etc.) to follow in His footsteps. There are too many needs around us for us to simply ignore.

Besides, as His Torch Bearers, God wants us to use the trials and challenges we face in life to help others. No one is immune from trouble. The issue is how we react to our challenges and difficulties. As a matter of fact, as Bishop T.D Jakes asserts that *'the more you're effective, the more you get into the hit list of hell... the closer you get to Jesus, the more the enemy gets intimidated'*. The devil only attacks those who cause him a lot of trouble. In my own case, the enemy thought he could threaten and intimidate me with cancer. Little did he know that God allowed it because He wanted to show the world what it is to be His True Torch Bearer. He wanted me to know that carrying the Olympic Torch was not the issue, but carrying the Torch of the Gospel and shining His light, in sickness and in health, was much more important.

Through the special grace of God, I had no problems whatsoever with my treatment. Sometimes I went for my radiotherapy treatment from work. At other times I would go for my treatment and then go to work from there. Even the letter from the Consultant Clinical Oncologist to my GP confirmed it all. She wrote *"treatment was completed as per protocol. The patient continued to work throughout her treatment and on the whole coped very well"*. This is a true testimony of God's faithfulness. I think the devil got more than he bargained for. He thought he would put my life on hold by threatening me with cancer, and not just the type of cancer that was common, but one that was rare and peculiar. However, he failed to realise that the power of our God within us is greater than his threats, and that *'we are more than conquerors'* through Christ. I am looking forward to the special pamper and spa treatment my family got for me, as their Mother's Day present. Glory to Jesus; that what the enemy meant for evil, God has turned it around for good, for His own glory.

No matter what we go through in life, there will always be others who are much worse off than ourselves. That was one thing that my own experience showed me. Every day that I walked into the NCCC, I saw people who were much worse off. In spite of what I was going through, I felt the pain of all those around me at that Centre. As true Torch Bearers, the Lord wants us to open our eyes to see the needs of people around us. We must pray and ask Him to make our hearts tender towards people; to help us never to miss the opportunity to be a blessing to someone EVERYDAY. We should go to bed every day with a smile on our face and gratitude in our hearts to God because we made a difference in some one's life that day. It could be just a smile. And in Matthew 25: 31- 46 the Bible tells us that on that day, the Lord Jesus would say to us *"Come, you blessed of My Father, inherit the kingdom prepared for you from the foundation of the world"*.

Be inspired...
Be challenged...
TRANSFORM YOUR LIFE

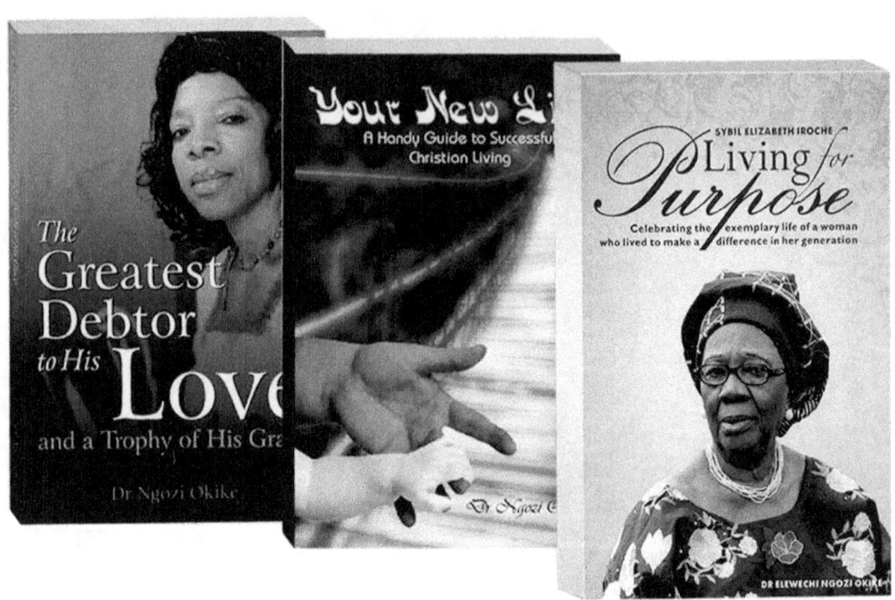

Be a winner...
Get your copy now!!!

**These books unlock the secrets to overcoming
Persecution • Life's Challenges • Impossibilities**

Available at www.amazon.co.uk; www.assurancepublications.com
or your local christian bookshop.

www.ingramcontent.com/pod-product-compliance
Lightning Source LLC
Chambersburg PA
CBHW061432050726
47593CB00006B/2320